RA
418
.5
.P6
. BET

Human Development Network
Health, Nutrition, and Population Series

Better Health Systems for India's Poor

Findings, Analysis, and Options

David H. Peters
Abdo S. Yazbeck
Rashmi R. Sharma
G. N. V. Ramana
Lant H. Pritchett
Adam Wagstaff

THE WORLD BANK
Washington, D.C.

a.IBRD/2002 (13)

Contents

Tables

Figures

Boxes

Foreword

What type of health system should India have in the 21st century?

That was the question posed by the government of India when it asked the World Bank to help analyze India's health system. The recognition was growing that conditions in India were changing rapidly, that the health system needed to keep up with these changes, and that important aspects of the health system were being overlooked by current approaches.

Through a wide consultative process that included many of India's internal and external development partners, a set of topics was selected for study, with results reviewed as they emerged. More than a dozen Indian institutions, in partnership with the World Bank and the Government of India, conducted the research. The studies provided new data and analysis that have not been available before on a number of fundamental issues of health care in India:

- The behavior of the private market in health

- The prevalence of chronic disease risk factors

- The distribution of benefits from different types of public and private health services

- The degree of financial protection in health care

- The degree of protection of patients' interests
- The laws and practices guiding health care.

Better Health Systems for India's Poor fills many gaps in understanding and synthesizes much about what can be learned from India's health system. Emerging from this analysis is an important set of principles for reform:

- Look after the health needs of the poor and vulnerable sections of society
- Prepare for the health transition with appropriate health financing systems and programs
- Harness the energy of the private sector while counteracting its failures
- Focus on quality and accountability in health services.

The key features of this work—the consultative processes, the sensitivity to variations in conditions among groups and regions, the clarity of analysis, and the tangibility of the alternatives for reform—make this study relevant to any country interested in making its health systems more effective, equitable, and accountable.

Jo Ritzen
Vice President
Human Development Network
The World Bank

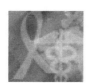

Preface

A host of questions emerged as the study team, assembled at the request of the government of India, considered the future of the Indian health care system. But throughout the consultations and deliberations, two questions remained foremost:

1. How can India meet the health needs of the most vulnerable segments of its population?

2. How can the roles of the public and private sectors be structured to better finance and deliver health services?

The overall aim of the exercise was to help India answer these questions, by informing and facilitating a professional and public discussion on the future directions for India's health system. This report synthesizes the resulting detailed studies that addressed different aspects of these questions. The report is intended for a variety of audiences, including policymakers, health sector managers and workers, researchers, consumer advocates, staff in development agencies, and the public interested in the health system and development in India. Representatives of these stakeholders were involved in the selection, design, conduct, and dissemination of the research summarized in this report.

In 1999, the research agenda for the studies was set through widespread consultations among many parties: central and state government officials, private sector providers, health insurance companies, not-for-profit providers, legal experts, academics, research groups, consumer organizations, medical associations, international agencies (World Health Organization, United Nations Children's Fund, European Union, Department for International Development—United Kingdom, and U.S. Agency for International Development), and experts within the World Bank. Small working groups were established to collaboratively prepare terms of reference for each study that was identified. The studies themselves were conducted by Indian institutions.

During 2000 and 2001, the same stakeholders were asked to go through the findings of the studies as they emerged and to formulate and discuss options. International experts and those in India also provided advice on the individual studies and this report.

The studies have produced data and analysis not previously available on several key topics: (a) the behavior of the private market in health, (b) the prevalence of chronic disease risk factors, (c) the distribution of benefits from different types of public and private health services, (d) the degree of financial protection in health, (e) schemes for the protection of patient interests, and (f) Indian law on health care. Appendix A lists the individual studies, the research organizations, the policy questions addressed, and use of study results. The 21 reports from the individual studies are listed as background papers in appendix B.

The studies are selective; they were not intended to cover all aspects of the Indian health system in detail, especially not aspects, such as public sector health services, on which considerable information was already available. In contrast, much research was conducted on the private sector, for which little information was available.

Moreover, the scope of the overall study itself was selective. Important sectors that influence health but that are not part of the direct delivery of health care—such as education, sanitation, and water supply—are not examined in detail in the report. Within the health sector, important issues concerning health manpower development and pharmaceutical policy were not studied in detail on the belief that analysis of these topics should be influenced by other choices about how the health system would be shaped.

The report focuses on four areas of the health system in which, in the judgment of the study group, reforms and innovations would make the most difference to the future of the Indian health system: oversight, public health service delivery, ambulatory curative care, and inpatient care, together with health insurance.

Part 1 of the report contains four chapters that discuss current conditions and policy options. Part 2 presents the theory and evidence to support the policy choices. The general reader may be most interested in the overview chapter and in the highlights found at the beginning of each of the chapters in part 2. These highlights outline the empirical findings and the main policy challenges discussed in the chapter.

If reforms are to be carried out in India's health sector, the vision for change must come out of the discussions among the stakeholders in the health system. Therefore, the report does not set out to prescribe detailed answers for India's future health system. It does, however, have a goal: to support informed debate and consensus building, and to help shape a health system that continually strives to be more effective, equitable, efficient, and accountable to the Indian people, and particularly to the poor.

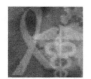

Acknowledgments

This report is a product of a wide range of consultations with policymakers, professional associations, academics, private sector representatives, and nongovernmental organizations (NGOs). Key findings were discussed at six workshops: one in Calcutta, through the State Health Systems Development Projects annual review; one in New Delhi, organized by the Voluntary Organization in the Interest of Consumer Organization; two in Hyderabad, organized by the Administrative Staff College of India; one in Lucknow, organized by the Indian Institute of Management; and in New Delhi, a final, national seminar organized with the Ministry of Health and Family Welfare. Active participation was received, with appreciation, from state Secretaries of Health, researchers, and other representatives of national and state governments, NGOs, consumer groups, and development agencies.

The teams that developed terms of reference for the background papers, and the authors of those papers themselves, made significant contributions to each others' work and to this final report; the authors of the papers included R. Baru, S. Chakraborty, G. Chellaraj, R. Durvasula, A. Ferreiro, C. Garg, R. Govindaraj, R. Kutty, A. Mahal, P. Mahapatra, B. Misra, V.R. Muraleedharan, S. Nandraj, M. Pearson, K. Prasad, R. Priya, I. Qadeer, K.S. Reddy, V. Selvaraju, P. Srivastava, A.J. Syed, A. Thekkuveetti, and S.K. Verma.

The extensive collaboration of the Government of India's Ministry of Health and Family Welfare, led by Mr. J. Chowdhury, Secretary, is acknowledged. Mr. K.K. Bakshi and Ms. Shailaja Chandra, initiated the studies while at the Ministry of Health and Family Welfare. Ms. K. Sujatha Rao, Joint Secretary, Ministry of Health and Family Welfare, spearheaded the organization of stakeholders and the three workshops and numerous meetings that helped shape the studies.

This report was prepared by a team led by David H. Peters. Abdo S. Yazbeck, Rashmi R. Sharma, and G.N.V. Ramana were full-time team members. Other team members were Lant H. Pritchett and Adam Wagstaff. Major contributions to the development of the studies were made by Richard Feacham and Monica Das Gupta.

Bruce Ross-Larson, Barbara Karni, Steve Kennedy, and Stephanie Rostron, all with Communications Development, assisted with the editing. For this publication, Gregg Forte edited the final product, with Janet H. Sasser serving as the production editor. Janmejay Singh, Pronita Chakrabarti, and Prasun Bhattacharjee provided research assistance. Particular thanks go to Nina Anand and Katia Gomes Pinto Visconti for administrative support and help with production of the report.

Richard Skolnik, in his capacity as Director, South Asia, Human Development, and Tawhid Nawaz, India Team Leader, worked closely with the team, which was also supported by the South Asia Health, Nutrition, and Population team and the India Country Team. The report is endorsed by Edwin Lim, India Country Director, and Joelle Chassard-Manibog, Country Coordinator.

The team was advised by Alexander S. Preker, April Harding, Philip Musgrove, Davidson Gwatkin, and Robert Fryatt. Also providing peer review were R. Radhakrishna, K.V. Narayana, P.S. Vashishtha, R. Bhatt, C.A.K. Yesudian, and P. Srinivasan. A quality enhancement review of the studies was conducted by Alain Colliou, Susan Stout, Shanta Devarajan, and Maureen Lewis. Substantive comments were made by the following colleagues from the World Bank: Mukesh Chawla, Edgardo Favaro, Jeffrey Hammer, Clive Harris, Peter F. Heywood, Manuel Jimenez, Sanjay Kathuria, Benjamin Loevinsohn, Anthony Measham, Tawhid Nawaz, Richard Skolnik, and Roberto Zagha. Numerous colleagues from outside the

Bank provided comments and suggestions at various stages of the work, including Cristian Baeza, Anne Bamasaiye, Victor Barbiero, Kevin Brown, Ken Grant, Indrani Gupta, Pradeep Kakkar, Tim Martineau, David Nicholas, J.-P. Poullier, Pravin Visaria, and M.S. Valiathan.

The preparation of the background papers and the convening of several workshops were supported by the Ministry of Health and Family Welfare, World Health Organization, Department for International Development—United Kingdom, U.S. Aid for International Development, the Dutch government, and the World Bank.

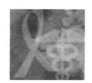

Acronyms and Abbreviations

AIDS	Acquired immune deficiency syndrome
AIIMS	All Indian Institute of Medical Sciences
ANM	Auxiliary nurse midwives
AP	Andhra Pradesh
APP	Alternative private practitioner
ASCI	Administrative Staff College of India
BAIF	Bharatiya Agro Industries Foundation
BMC	Bombay Municipal Corporation
CAG	Citizen, Consumer and Civic Action Group
CEHAT	Centre for Enquiry into Health and Allied Themes
CBHI	Central Bureau of Health Intelligence
CGHS	Central Government Health Scheme
CHC	Community Health Centre
CPR	Centre for Policy Research
CSS	Centre for Social Studies
DALY	Disability-adjusted life year
DFID	Department for International Development
DHS	Demographic and health surveys
DOTS	Directly observed treatment short-course
ESIS	Employees State Insurance Scheme
EU	European Union
GIC	General Insurance Corporation
GDP	Gross domestic product
GHIP	Group Health Insurance Program

GP	General practitioner
HAP	Health Action for the People
HIV	Human immunodeficiency virus
HNP	Health, Nutrition, and Population (The World Bank)
ICDS	Integrated Child Development Services
IEG	Institute of Economic Growth
IHBAS	Institute of Human Behavior and Allied Sciences
IMR	Infant mortality rate
IHD	Institute for Human Development
IHS	Institute of Health Systems
IIPS	Indian Institute for Population Sciences
ISM	Indian Systems of Medicine
JSS	Jagadguru Sri Shivarathreeshwara (College of Pharmacy)
MBBS	Bachelor of Medicine and Bachelor of Surgery
MGRMU	The Tamil Nadu Dr. M. G. R. Medical University
MOHFW	Ministry of Health and Family Welfare
MTP	Medical termination of pregnancy
NCAER	National Council for Applied Economic Research
NGO	Nongovernmental organization
NIPFP	National Institute of Public Finance and Policy
NTP	National Tuberculosis Control Programs
NSSO	National Sample Survey Organisation
PHC	Primary health center
PRI	Panchayati Raj Institution
SC/ST	Scheduled caste or tribe
STD	Sexually transmitted disease
STEM	Center for Symbiosis of Technology, Environment and Management
TRIPS	Trade-related aspects of intellectual property
TB	Tuberculosis
TFR	Total fertility rate
UNICEF	United Nations Children's Fund
UP	Uttar Pradesh
USAID	U.S. Agency for International Development
WHO	World Health Organization

Overview

India's health system is at a crossroads. Since the country's Independence, in 1947, India's health conditions have changed. A high proportion of the population continues to suffer and die from preventable infections, pregnancy and childbirth-related complications, and undernutrition. At the same time, new health threats are stretching the capacity of the health system to respond. An estimated 3.5 million Indians are living with human immunodeficiency virus (HIV), and the virus has now spread beyond highly susceptible groups to the general population in some states, threatening to erase much of the social, economic, and health gains since Independence. Also besetting the population now are noncommunicable diseases such as heart disease and mental illness, health problems associated with countries with a higher income than India. Building robust health systems requires building the capacity to do better on the "unfinished agenda" of health problems as well as meet the emerging realities and challenges.

India is in the midst of a "health transition"—at varying rates depending on the state and population group. The transition is demographic— a decline in mortality and fertility rates and an aging of the population; epidemiological—a shift in the pattern of ill health from malnutrition and communicable disease to the chronic diseases of adulthood; and social—rising capabilities and expectations of the population regarding health care. A high proportion of the population continues, however, to suffer and die from preventable infections, pregnancy and childbirth-related complications, and undernutrition—the "unfinished agenda" of the health transition. The large disparities across India place the burden of these conditions mostly on the poor, women, and scheduled tribes and castes. The poorest 20 percent of Indians, for example, have more than double the mortality rates, malnutrition, and fertility of the richest quintile.

Despite all this, the public remains uninformed about much of the health system. It knows little about whether health services are appropriate, who is benefiting from them, whether quality is sufficient, or whether people are getting good value from public and private spending on health. Equity, quality, and accountability are badly wanting in both the public and private health sectors. The time has come to reassess how the Indian health system should function and to retool it for the new millennium.

This report is a product of extensive consultations and research conducted by more than a dozen Indian institutions. The report does not propose a blueprint for reform. The experience that emerged from its preparation strongly suggests that vision, broadly based political work, and a spirit of experimentation, rather than an abstract plan, are the key ingredients of any future improvements; plans and projects that do not emerge from a collaborative process animated by such ingredients will not be meaningful. The report clearly shows that reform is needed, however, and it outlines some broad principles for reform efforts, which should be led by government. The main message is that the government and the public should raise their sights in four ways:

1. Take responsibility for the needs of the entire population—by making the health system more pro-poor, gender sensitive, and client friendly, and by responding to the high burden of preventable diseases borne by the poor, scheduled tribes and castes, and women.

2. Look forward to the health transition—by preparing for the shift in disease burden and increase in health costs by developing health financing systems.

3. Remove the blind spot to the private sector—by harnessing its energy and countering its failures.

4. Focus efforts—by emphasizing quality, efficiency, and accountability of health services in both public and private sectors.

Ultimately, changing the shape of the health system depends on political decisions at national, state, and local levels—decisions that will be shaped by expressions of political preferences, social expectations, and the positions that leaders take at each level. International experience tells us that no single correct answer can be found for shaping a country's health system. In India, the priority of issues and choice of options should vary according to the conditions in the various states and districts. An explicit approach to policy formulation and implementation will help to continually evolve the health system—and to ensure that the health system is improving the health of all Indians in an accountable, equitable, and affordable manner.

The Indian Health System

Despite the establishment of a large public network of health providers, public spending on health is very low, stagnant at around 1 percent of gross domestic product (GDP). Such spending puts India among the bottom 20 percent of countries. It is lower than what most low-income countries spend, and it is far below what is needed to provide basic health care to the population. The large variance in health financing among Indian states is increasing the gap in public resources for health between rich and poor states; and it threatens to expand existing gaps in health system outcomes. The states of Kerala, Punjab, and Tamil Nadu, for example, have double the per capita public health spending of Bihar and Madhya Pradesh.

As in other countries, public spending on preventive health services has a lower priority than curative care. And curative services themselves are highly pro-rich in distribution. About 3 rupees (Rs) is spent on the richest quintile for every Rs 1 spent on the poorest 20 percent (figure O.1). Yet in three states (Kerala, Tamil Nadu, and Maharashtra), the distribution of public spending on health is nearly

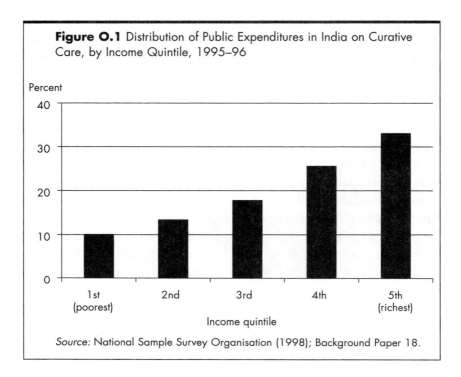

Figure O.1 Distribution of Public Expenditures in India on Curative Care, by Income Quintile, 1995–96

Percent

Source: National Sample Survey Organisation (1998); Background Paper 18.

uniform across income groups. Statistically, states with better equality in their public spending have better health status outcomes.

Private health spending presents a different story. It accounts for more than 80 percent of all health spending, one of the highest proportions of private spending found anywhere in the world. Nearly all the private spending in India is out-of-pocket at the point of service use, an inefficient way to finance health care that leaves people highly vulnerable. As in most developing countries, poorer households purchase less curative health care from the private sector than do richer households. Partly because of inability to pay and the lack of risk pooling, the poor are much less likely to be hospitalized. Across India, those above the poverty line have more than double the hospitalization rates of the poor.

Hospitalization frequently results in financial catastrophe, especially in the absence of risk-pooling mechanisms. Only 10 percent of Indians have some form of insurance, and most of the forms are

inadequate. Hospitalized Indians spent 58 percent of their total
annual expenditures on health care. More than 40 percent of hospitalized people borrow money or sell assets to cover expenses. One
conservative estimate finds that one-fourth of hospitalized Indians
were not poor when they entered the hospital but became so because
of hospital expenses, a risk that, like many other elements of the
Indian health system, varies greatly from state to state (figure O.2).

Even at public hospitals, which are intended to protect the poor
from financial risks, the poor are vulnerable to health costs. Indeed, in
some states (Uttar Pradesh, West Bengal, Madhya Pradesh, Rajasthan,
Haryana, and Bihar), the poor are more likely to borrow money when
hospitalized in the public sector than in the private sector.

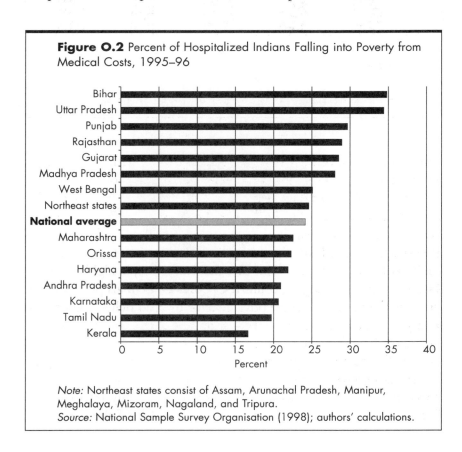

Figure O.2 Percent of Hospitalized Indians Falling into Poverty from
Medical Costs, 1995–96

Note: Northeast states consist of Assam, Arunachal Pradesh, Manipur,
Meghalaya, Mizoram, Nagaland, and Tripura.
Source: National Sample Survey Organisation (1998); authors' calculations.

The private sector accounts for the majority of curative care services in India, although, again, considerable variation exists across services and states (figure O.3). Overall, the distribution of services in the private sector is even more skewed toward the rich than it is in the public sector. The poor still depend on the public sector for the majority of their health services, with one exception—the private sector provides 79 percent of outpatient care for those below the poverty line, much of which is of low quality and provided by untrained practitioners.

An important group of providers are the alternative private practitioners, consisting of two groups: one, those who attempt to practice Western, allopathic medicine without training in the discipline; and the other, those who practice Indian systems of medicine. The alternative private practitioners make up a larger segment of the private ambulatory care market than qualified allopathic doctors. Regardless of type of provider, quality assurance is a problem, with most care reflecting poor clinical practices and standards and inadequate staffing. Many opportunities are, however, identified in this report for the government to work with or influence the practice of private providers, including simple measures to help improve the quality of the care from alternative private practitioners.

The large variation between states—a major theme of this report—means that recommendations for the whole of India or even for groups of states run the risk of oversimplification (table O.1 shows one categorization of states used in this report). Health is a shared responsibility of the central government and the states. How much discretion each state has over the policy options in any given area will vary. In some public health activities, the central government will likely take the lead through centrally sponsored schemes. But in curative services, states already exhibit enormous variations in what they do and in how well they do it; and vulnerable groups are affected differently in the various states. Such findings substantiate the need to look at solutions that are specific to different conditions in the states and that address several areas of the health system. The new areas of analysis show important differences and the particular vulnerability of the poor in:

Figure O.3 Public and Private Sector Shares of Delivery of Selected Health Care Services in India, by Income Status of Patients, 1995–96

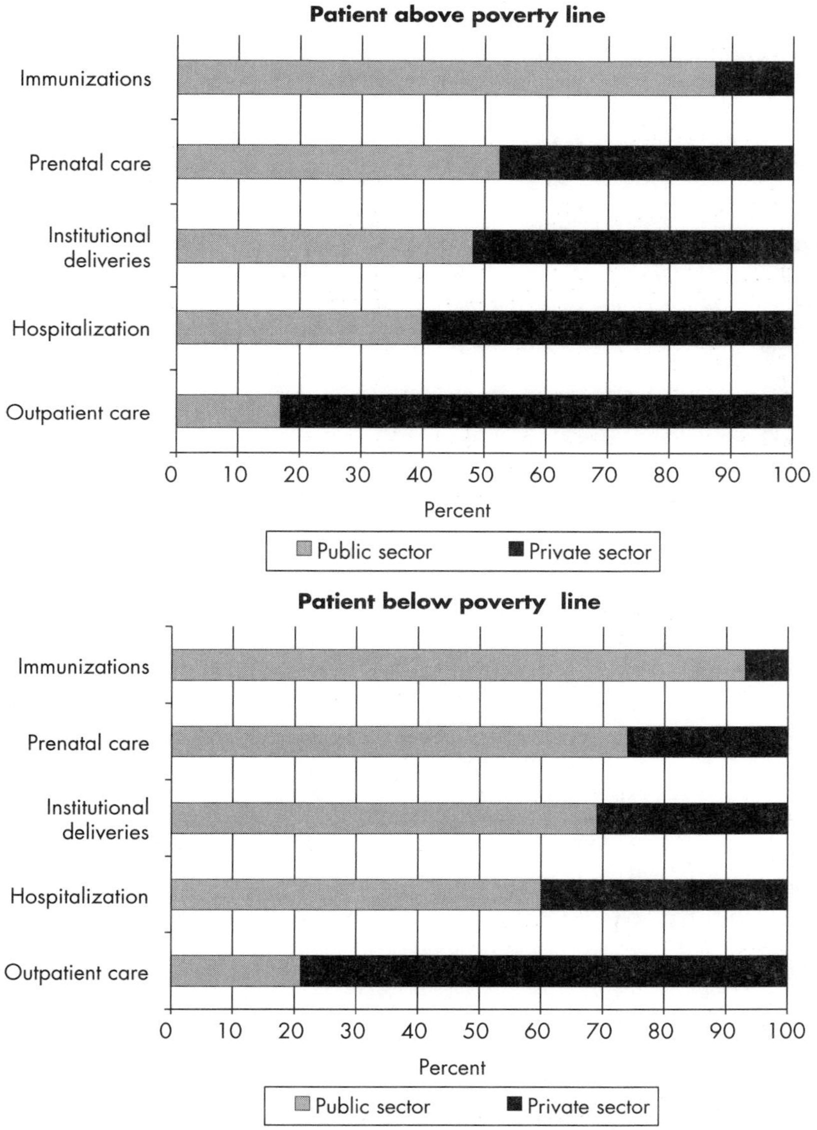

Patient above poverty line

Patient below poverty line

Source: National Sample Survey Organisation (1998); authors' calculations.

Table O.1 Major Indian States, by Stage of Health Transition and Institutional Capacity

STAGE OF TRANSITION, DEGREE OF CAPACITY	STATES	INDIA'S POPULATION (PERCENT)
Middle to late transition, moderate to high capacity	Kerala, Tamil Nadu	9.1
Early to middle transition, low to moderate capacity	Maharashtra, Karnataka, Punjab, West Bengal, Andhra Pradesh, Gujarat, Haryana	39.1
Very early transition, very low to low capacity	Orissa, Rajasthan, Madhya Pradesh, Uttar Pradesh	33.1
Special cases: instability, high to very high mortality, civil conflict, poor governance	Assam, Bihar	13.3

Note: Major Indian states are those with a population of at least 15 million. The estimates were made before bifurcation, so Bihar includes the recently created state of Jharkhand, Madhya Pradesh includes Chatisgarh, and Uttar Pradesh includes Uttaranchal.

- The behavior of the private market in health (chapter 6)
- The prevalence of chronic disease risk factors (chapter 7)
- The distribution of public and private health services (chapter 7)
- The degree of financial protection in health (chapters 8 and 9)
- The protection of patients' interests (chapter 9).

Which Way Forward?

The first four chapters of the report analyze the policy context and the choices for different activities, states, and programs. The focus is on strategies for four critical sets of activities selected from the larger set of functions of the health system. These strategies are summarized in the set of tables—"Options at a Glance"—at the end of this overview.

a. Health system oversight

b. Public health service delivery

c. Ambulatory curative services

d. Inpatient care and health financing.

Although changes will also be needed in the management of other inputs to the health system—such as human resource development, pharmaceuticals, technology development and assessment, and knowledge management—this report does not concentrate on them. But actions in those areas should support decisions made in the four critical areas of activity just listed.

Oversight

One of the main gaps in India's health system is in oversight. As a clear "public good" that benefits all persons, oversight is an area that requires public action. The analysis in this report demonstrates that increasing the measurability of health care providers and other actors is sorely needed. Example of activities that will increase measurability are collecting and analyzing information on price, type, and volume of cases and on service-quality indicators such as the use of technology and clinical outcomes. One of the most important considerations for the central government is whether it will spend more effort on overseeing the health sector, perhaps at the expense of directly managing public sector service delivery.

The financial costs of strengthening oversight are small, and the benefits are considerable. Oversight activities are a prerequisite to improving quality, equity, and being able to use health insurance or strategic purchasing of health services. But public action is not synonymous with government action. One cannot assume that creating a government body with responsibilities and powers of oversight over the health sector will improve matters. Public oversight means empowering people who use the health system. Therefore, a wider variety of potential actions to improve oversight are considered.

The growing prominence of the private sector makes the development of oversight by the public sector more urgent than ever. International and domestic experiences suggest, however, that relying on only one approach to such oversight is unlikely to be sufficient. Considering the almost nonexistent formal collaboration to date between the public and private sectors and the public sector's limited enforcement of regulations, the most productive strategies are likely to be those that take a balanced approach. Each state ought to develop its own policies and strategies and then engage the private sector in developing a common agenda. Using independent organizations as honest brokers to measure performance may also be a better way to start than relying on government or provider organizations, because the problems of credibility and conflict may be larger at the beginning of these reforms.

But such steps also depend on the development of trust between public and private sector players, which can also be enhanced through the involvement of professional organizations. Increasing the role of consumer advocates is another good approach to strengthening oversight, particularly to make health services more directly accountable to the public. Formal public sector regulation will still be needed, but the analysis suggests that these approaches have more potential to be more successful in regulating factor inputs to the health sector, such as drug quality control, than they do in regulating provider and hospital behaviors. In any case, given the limitations in public sector regulatory capacity, it is best to be selective in starting actions to strengthen formal public regulation.

States in the middle to later stages of the health transition and with moderate to high institutional capacity can use these strategies to institutionalize quality assurance procedures in inpatient and ambulatory services. States earlier in the transition and with less capacity may have to focus initial activities on expanding public information approaches to empower people to demand better health services—and on initiating steps to bring public and private sector actors together. As states gain experience and confidence, they can pursue more options.

Public Health Service Delivery

Public health services considered here are the programs and institutions organized by society that directly protect, promote, and restore peoples' health through collective action. As with oversight activities, these services are "public goods" or have significant benefits beyond the individual, giving strong justification for government involvement. Some of the main challenges facing public health are:

- How can India best fight the HIV/AIDS (acquired immune deficiency syndrome) epidemic?

- How can critical gaps be removed in planning, implementation, monitoring, technical leadership, and communications?

- How can programs for existing public health priorities be strengthened, while decentralizing responsibilities and resources to states?

- When and how should effective programs be developed to address emerging public health priorities, such as the health consequences of smoking, mental illness, and injuries?

Because India invests so little in public health, both in relative and absolute terms, the most relevant actions involve allocating more resources and effort on public health services. However, simply putting more money into public health will not be sufficient.

Most of India is still in the early part of the health transition, so it should redouble its efforts to attack the unfinished agenda as its highest public health priority. The success of public health programs usually depends on more than funding the technical interventions, as demonstrated in recent success stories in health in low-income countries. In the short term, intensive training and supervision in management, provision of supplies, and stronger and more professional health education that strengthens people's ability to make healthy choices are important measures to make these programs more effective. Continuing the current approaches across the country is unlikely to suffice, however, even with additional resources. The evidence from our studies makes a convincing case to involve private practitioners in these critical programs in most states because of their extensive reach and willingness to participate.

Differences among states must be recognized and considered. Kerala and Tamil Nadu, being further along in the transition and having greater capacity, have more compelling reasons to focus on introducing and expanding public health services for cardiovascular disease, mental health, and injuries, as these are now the prominent conditions facing their populations. Other states are earlier in the transition but should also consider selective interventions in these areas. For example, Orissa and West Bengal have very high rates of tobacco use, particularly among their poor. They should consider putting more effort into public health campaigns against tobacco, and ensure that they are not using public funds to subsidize or encourage tobacco production and use.

All states need to place additional effort on HIV prevention because of the disease's potential for damage and the need for timely action, although the balance of interventions may be different from state to state because of differences in social conditions and transmission patterns. The HIV epidemic and the emergence of other diseases have also exposed the weaknesses of the current public health system. In the medium to long term, investing in public health systems is a necessary strategy to provide the personnel and systems needed to carry out the current agenda and respond to future challenges.

Ambulatory Curative Services

The major challenges in service provision are fourfold: improving quality, increasing accountability, controlling costs, and promoting equity. These challenges raise several questions:

- Can government effectively purchase services from the private sector?

- Can performance and costs in the private and public sectors be properly monitored?

- Can government further extend coverage of health services to the poor by encouraging and perhaps formalizing pro-poor measures now being provided by the private sector?

- Can government effectively monitor health gains by the poor?

- How can India balance the dual challenges of expanding public spending on critical health services and improving regional equity in resource allocation?

- How can the experience of stronger states be replicated in poorly performing states to improve health status and reduce polarization?

Some clear choices face governments in the area of ambulatory care. Economic analysis indicates that outpatient care is the area in which the rationale for direct government provision of services is weakest. Two countervailing facts, however, are that (a) many preventive health programs depend on the opportunities and infrastructure used for outpatient curative care, and (b) outpatient care is the area in which the public has the most contact with the health system and where most private money is spent. Outpatient care is therefore a public concern, at least from an oversight perspective. The options considered here all involve relatively more resources than oversight and public health actions, although room may exist for better use of the large amount of private money already being spent on ambulatory care.

Given the large presence of the private sector, all states clearly need to focus more attention on services provided privately. Supporting the oversight options can help to do this. But it also means delivering more credible ambulatory care services through both public and private sectors. The report explores many options for doing so.

Influencing private practice by financing them and focusing public delivery on areas where the private sector does not reach should be the most logical choices for most states. In states with low institutional capacity, high infant mortality, and low coverage of basic public health measures (such as for immunizations and nutrition), a reduction in publicly provided ambulatory curative care would allow a reallocation of effort into public health activities. The most expensive option is to try to revitalize the entire network of public facilities. Following such a strategy without a several-fold increase in resources may avoid difficult political decisions, but it would lead to little improvement in public services. The resources are spread too thinly, and efforts to improve availability and performance of staff and other resources have made slow progress. Even if a windfall of resources were to become available, strategies would still be needed to deal with the much larger private sector that is preferred by the majority of the Indians.

Inpatient Care and Financing

For inpatient care and financing, some of the same challenges identified for ambulatory care are also relevant when considering quality, costs, accountability, and equity.

- How can India as a whole learn from its better-performing states and address regional equality in resource allocation?

- How can the distribution of public expenditures be improved so that a greater fraction reaches the poor?

- How will India take on the task of moving from out-of-pocket, fee-for-service financing to risk-pooling mechanisms in a weak regulatory environment?

- How can public and private health facilities be made more responsive to the needs of their clients?

- Can client perceptions of providers' manners and skills be incorporated in training and supervision programs to make health providers more responsive?

- Can governments intervene in areas that would make the biggest difference in motivating health workers, notably training opportunities?

Some unique challenges also face this segment of the health system. Inpatient care is particularly expensive and risky. A "two-tier" system may emerge in which the poor are effectively left out of quality care in the public sector (due to low access and quality) and the private sector (due to cost). Plans for care or insurance that attempt to provide the poor with exactly the same quality and quantity of inpatient care as the rich receive run the risk of cost escalation.

Because of the close relationship between financing and high-cost-per-episode inpatient care, we consider sets of options for financing and provision of inpatient care together. The reforms proposed are not cheap, but the costs of not reforming are even greater. Given the high levels of private financing and debt currently caused by inpatient care, methods that are able to capture some of this funding while preventing the hardships of the current situation will have a greater chance of long-term success.

India needs to set its sights on developing a more efficient and equitable health financing system. This means a financing system that has compulsory membership, a socially acceptable and affordable package of benefits, pre-payment, and risk pooling for people with different incomes and health status. The main questions are when and how to get there. Progress is likely to come from those states with the greatest administrative capacity and whose governments are able to learn from the experimental and smaller-scale community financing schemes being tested by some NGOs. Big experiments are particularly needed to see how to cover the large informal sector, and to gain positive experience in managing health insurance.

Relying on private health insurance is likely to play some role in the short term, since the insurance market has been liberalized, and this consumes little additional public resources. But the central government will probably have to play a more aggressive role in regulating private insurance. International experience has shown that the cost of not tightly regulating private voluntary health insurance is that regulating it later on will become more necessary because of escalating health costs and increased inequalities, yet more difficult to do because private interests will have become more entrenched and practices more firmly established.

Pursuing options for reform of hospital provision are complementary to those oriented around financing. For states earlier in the transition and with less capacity, the most reasonable approach would be for governments to spend more effort on improving the quality of existing public first-referral hospitals, but to do so in a selective manner that promotes more equitable distribution of public resources. Experience has shown that such approaches can lead to improved quality of care and greater efficiencies, although only after several years.

*****

In conclusion, now is the time to conduct big experiments throughout India's health care system, particularly since the status quo is leading to a dead end. Either the central government or individual states could take the initiative, but new experience is needed to build on what has become an outmoded health system. The opportunity exists now for governments to reform the way they work—and to take on critical oversight functions. Governments also need to consider new public health services and how to implement them in ways that improve on current approaches. New ways of managing ambulatory and inpatient services should also be tried, along with a concerted effort to develop a more efficient, equitable, and risk-reducing health financing system.

The new experiments need flexibility if they are to deal with the highly varied conditions found across India, and they must include intensive monitoring and evaluation if lessons are to be learned. Clearly, no single choice is best for India. But the broadest opportunity exists now—to travel with eyes open, consciously deciding which fork in the road to take. Those who seek the right way must consult, analyze, debate, and forge a consensus on key issues and be willing to try new options. In the long run, this approach will best enable India's health system to meet the health needs of its people.

Options at a Glance

Table O.2 Improving Health System Oversight

ACTION	DESCRIPTION
1. Develop partnerships with private sector to share information, improve quality, and cooperate on service provision	Build networks of private and public providers; seek cooperation on information, materials, training; and use tools such as subsidies and contracting. These activities could have relatively low financial costs and offer the possibility of improving efficiency and increasing service coverage without adding staff to the government. Contracting offers the prospect of increasing accountability and creating efficiencies that could not be attained with direct government provision of services.
2. Support independent organizations to measure performance in public and private sectors	Provide an honest broker capable of better resisting unwanted pressures from the public and private sector. The broker might also be more efficient.
3. Facilitate health-advocacy organizations independent of both public providers and private associations to work as consumer advocates	Simulate new organizations to become more active representatives of people's concerns in the health sector. Such organizations hold the promise of greater participation by people in their health care, and could help raise accountability and performance of health services at relatively low costs.
4. Support professional self-regulation	Use professional bodies to more actively regulate practitioners through measures such as continuing medical education, accreditation of providers and facilities, and providing means for redress of patient complaints. Self-regulation is likely to be more attractive to service providers than regulation by the public sector.
5. Strengthen formal regulation of health inputs (drug quality)	Strengthen government agencies to regulate health inputs such as pharmaceuticals. Such organizations exist but are underfinanced, poorly organized, and poorly functioning.
6. Formalize public sector regulation of private providers	Create or strengthen government agencies responsible for the regulation of health care providers to set standards, license providers, receive complaints against providers, inspect premises, and generally take responsibility for bringing the private sector under public sector control.

17

Table O.3 Strengthening Public Health Services

ACTIONS	DESCRIPTION
1. Concentrate effort on programs for the "unfinished agenda" by: a. Increasing funding *and*	Allocate more resources to programs that combat the conditions of the unfinished agenda, namely diseases of childhood and maternity, malnutrition, tuberculosis, and malaria.
b. Increasing effectiveness	Focus activities on supervision, monitoring results, increasing public accountability, using professional communications strategies, strengthening logistics systems, training, decentralization, improvement of public health systems, and partnerships with the private sector.
2. Initiate and strengthen programs in non-communicable diseases in states well advanced in the epidemiological transition	Accelerate preventive interventions against cardiovascular and tobacco-related illnesses and develop more comprehensive programs to prevent injury and disability from major mental illness.
3. Reduce centrally sponsored schemes, turn over the resources to the states, reassign functions of the central Ministry of Health and Family Welfare	Refocus functions of the central health ministry on developing policies and plans, allocating funds strategically, and sharing experiences and technical expertise, while devolving management of programs and institutions to the states and autonomous institutions. Centrally sponsored schemes might still be used for experimental activities (for example, the introduction of a public health insurance program), for programs of national interest in which public and political awareness is insufficient to ensure adequate attention (HIV control), and for states experiencing special hardships.
4. Reinvest heavily in public health systems generally	Invest in public health and health management training broadly, health information systems, disease surveillance, public health monitoring, and health promotion activities, as proposed by the Bajaj Commission (Bajaj 1996).

18

Table O.4 Strengthening Ambulatory Curative Services

ACTION	DESCRIPTION
1. Focus public resources strategically by	
a. Revitalizing the network of public sector facilities in disadvantaged areas	Be selective and focus on raising the quality of public sector facilities in poor areas and where NGO and qualified private sector providers have not been forthcoming; do not try to cover the whole country or all rural areas with rigid input- and population-based norms.
and	
b. Purchasing curative care from the private sector when possible, limiting public provision from primary health centers (PHCs) and subcenters in those areas	Move critical functions such as prenatal care and family planning to public procurement via private sector providers, at least where quality private sector providers exist. Subsidize care for the poor.
2. Expand coverage for the poor through the use of demand-side mechanisms that give the poorest access to publicly subsidized discounts at either public or certified private providers	Build on existing mechanisms whereby private providers provide, or claim to provide, discounts to poorer customers. Offer direct reimbursement to certified private providers for services provided to poor clients, preferably through mechanisms that allow clients a choice among providers.
or	
3. Revitalize the entire network of public sector facilities to raise the quality of publicly provided services	Put money into public sector ambulatory care, notably care delivered at subcenters and PHCs across-the-board and make organizational and management changes to improve efficiency and public responsiveness.

19

Table O.5 Inpatient Care and Health Insurance

ACTIONS	DESCRIPTION
Financing-Oriented Alternatives:	
1. Encourage multiple insurance pools. Facilitate private insurance to pay private providers in a regulatory environment that encourages voluntary employer- or union-based insurance schemes, with public insurance schemes for the poor	Use competing private and social insurance systems to reach all with compulsory purchase of insurance, but with choices and public subsidies and equalization funds to cover the poorest. Takes advantage of multiple revenue raising mechanisms; but depends on development of quality assurance and information systems to distinguish good quality care from bad and strong ability to monitor and regulate.
or	
2. Initiate compulsory purchase of "single payer" insurance coverage	Develop publicly accountable universal health insurance that raises revenues publicly and maintains public and private provision and patient choice but also uses quality assurance and health information systems. Offers the ability to control costs, is easier to administer and regulate than other health insurance, and is a powerful way to align clinical practices with public priorities.
or	
3. Rely on the introduction of private voluntary health insurance	Continue the present course, whereby the wealthy obtain private insurance and health costs and inequities grow. Richer households are using public hospitals less and relying on private hospitals more, a trend that is fueling demand for private health insurance targeted primarily to wealthier households. As richer households abandon the public system, political support for public financing erodes. This could lead to a vicious circle in which low and deteriorating quality in the public sector drives middle- and high-income households into the private market, undermining public hospitals.
Provision-Oriented Alternatives:	
4. Invest in quality of care, especially in public sector secondary hospitals serving	Introducing quality improvements in underutilized public secondary hospitals increases their efficiency while providing services largely to the poor. This approach is popular among state

20

rural areas, but increase cost recovery with or without prepayment mechanisms to improve equality

bureaucracies and politicians, so ownership is high and implementation relatively good. By providing a small but important amount of funds for improving quality, cost recovery at such institutions becomes more politically and socially acceptable.

5. Make public hospitals autonomous, and fund their services publicly

Separates public sector "provision of insurance" from "provision of curative care." The revenues for these autonomous hospitals could be based strictly on reimbursement for care provided via a public sector financing mechanism—but with no explicit insurance premium, as costs would be paid from general revenues. Would also require careful monitoring of quality and social mandates to provide care to the poor.

PART 1

Raising the Sights for India's Health System

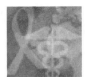

CHAPTER 1

A Crossroads

India's health system is at a crossroads. Its ability to fight infant mortality, communicable disease, and malnutrition is being stretched at the same time that it faces emerging demands for better service and more attention to the chronic diseases of adulthood. India's underfunded public sector and its extensively used but largely unaccountable private sector cannot hope to meet the country's enormous, growing, and shifting health needs. If India continues on its present path, the mismatch between its health system and its health problems will become only more severe. The present moment is a decisive one because the government of India is now seeking to define a better health system for the country, one that can take better advantage of the capacity of the private sector and deliver better service and outcomes for all regions and socioeconomic groups.

The overall state of health in India has been improving—life expectancy at birth rose from 49 years in 1970 to 63 years in 1998. But its historic health problems—among them high infant mortality, child malnourishment and its associated diseases, and high fertility—remain unresolved. For example, from the 1950s to 1990, infant mortality was halved, to about 70 deaths per 1,000 live births; but that rate is still too high and has moved little in the past decade. Also, childhood malnutrition and maternal health problems are still widespread—nearly half of children under five years of age are malnourished, while anemia afflicts about three-fourths of children under three and about half of women of reproductive age. And although India's national program for population control, launched in 1951, was one of the first in the world and met with some success, the 1999 fertility rate of 3.3 remains higher than in most other Asian countries. These problems—along with the communicable diseases of tuberculosis, malaria, and leprosy—constitute the unfinished agenda of the post-Independence health system.

Now added to the unfinished health agenda is a vast new threat. The human immunodeficiency virus (HIV) and its product, the autoimmune deficiency syndrome (AIDS), is spreading fast in India. With 3.5 million Indians already living with HIV, and with the virus in some states having spread beyond the most susceptible groups, the epidemic threatens to erase much of the social, economic, and health gains India has made since 1947, much as the disease is already turning back the clock in Sub-Saharan Africa.

This study finds that India's past success and current struggles together suggest new choices for its health system, both for government and for the private sector.

- Where should government focus its efforts—on the poor? On selective diseases, programs, or functions? On developing health financing systems?

- In what direction should the private sector be guided—toward outpatient care? Toward hospital care? Toward public service?

Although progress has stalled, the very social, economic, and health gains India has realized in the past 50 years have helped prepare the ground for the shift in health conditions that is emerging in India—the incipient "health transition." The health transition encompasses three specific and interrelated shifts: (a) demographic—a decline in rates of mortality and fertility and an aging of the population, (b) epidemiological—a change in the dominant pattern of disease, from malnutrition and the communicable diseases of childhood to the chronic diseases of adulthood, and (c) social—a general rise in knowledge and expectations of the health system and a greater ability to care for oneself. The health transition presents challenges unfamiliar to India, to be sure. But their solution may point the way to a new and more successful health system, one that can solve old problems while attending to the new. If India builds a health system that renews progress on the traditional health agenda, it must do so in a way that will also attend to the new health conditions and expectations that will come even faster with such success.

Objectives of the Health System and the Health Transition

A health system has three main objectives:

- Improve the *health status* of the population by lowering mortality and morbidity rates

- Protect the population against the *financial risks* of health problems

- Respond to *citizens' demands and needs*.

The relative importance of these objectives shifts as the health status and other conditions of a country improve and evolve. That shift constitutes the health transition that is now emerging in India even as it struggles with the stagnation of its health status.

When mortality is high and morbidity widespread, the primary objective is to improve life expectancy and health status by reducing avoidable health losses from malnutrition and from communicable and readily prevented or treated diseases of maternity, birth, and childhood. As progress is made on these conditions and in the basic infrastructure of public health services, as is happening in some areas of India, the three elements of the transition—demographic, epidemiological, and social—will alter the types of care required of the health system, raise the financial burden of disease, and increase the sensitivity of the system to social demands.

The demographic and epidemiological transitions: as rudimentary public health (water, sanitation, nutrition) improves and low-cost-per-episode conditions (diarrhea, respiratory infections, malaria) are better treated, the population ages and an increasing fraction of the disease burden and of health expenditures will come from high-cost-per-episode diseases. Besides presenting medical challenges, the new risk factors and diseases raise the *financial* vulnerability of the population and thereby challenge the health system's ability to protect individuals in that dimension as well.

The social transition: as the severity of pre-transition health conditions diminishes, the responsiveness of the system to citizens' demands and needs comes into sharper focus. The quality of health services—both technical and perceived—tends to become increasingly important as basic health conditions are addressed and expectations are raised.

Of particular concern in India is ensuring that, in pursuing each of the three objectives, the interests of the poor are protected. This concern does not mean that public health services ought to be made available only to the poor; in fact, the emerging "two-track" health care system, in which the poor can afford to use only the public sector hospitals of lower quality while the rich can afford to choose the better-performing hospitals, which are usually in the private sector, may be the *least* effective way to protect the poor. Neither the public nor the private system can be considered acceptable until it addresses the large gaps in outcomes between the poor and rich on each of the three objectives.

The Current Policy Context

India's current health policy has its origins in the nation-building activities at the time of Independence and in the thinking embodied in the Bhore Committee report (Bhore, Amesur, and Banerjee 1946). The Bhore Committee focused on primary health care (at that time seen as simple curative and preventive care that could be provided in a clinic or home setting); it laid down the principle that access to primary care is a basic right and thus not contingent on ability to pay or on any other socioeconomic condition. The commission established primary health care as the foundation of the national health care system and developed the first system for primary health care facilities and health personnel in the public sector. Building on this thinking, India became a strong supporter of the Alma Ata Declaration of 1978, in which it committed itself to attaining "Health For All" on the basis of the primary health care approach.

The Bhore Committee clearly modeled its vision for a public national health service on the one adopted by the United Kingdom (Bhore, Amesur, and Banerjee 1946). The early planners focused on a public national health service in part because the private sector involved with Western medicine was very small at that time. The vision was similar to the existing nationalization ideology of the United Kingdom. The approach in India was unlike that of high-income former British colonies such as Canada and Australia. By the end of World War II, those countries had large private sectors; they were able to guarantee universal access to health services through more pluralistic health systems.

Health policy in India has thus paid little attention to the private sector, though in recent years it has started to give it more consideration (see appendix C for a digest of national policy reports since Independence). By the time that India adopted its first formal national health policy, in 1983, the central government had recognized the need to "cooperate" with the private sector. Since then, however, efforts in that direction have been limited. The time has surely come to examine more specifically and seriously what can be done with the private health sector in India.

Historic Vision and Current Realities

Plans and policy options should be ambitious, but they should also be informed by the realities of the present. The vision of a universal, vertically integrated, publicly provided health care system has a utopian appeal. It holds out the promise of capturing synergies by linking preventive and promotional activities through ambulatory and inpatient clinical care; of improving quality and generating cost savings from an integrated referral chain that prevents routine cases from being treated in high-cost facilities; and of providing universal and equal coverage for all.

Indeed, after the Second World War, the comprehensive, universal approach was pursued in many countries in Europe and in former colonial areas of Africa and Asia. Over time, only countries that have had the political and social support for such systems have been able to maintain the high levels of public investment in health (more than 5 percent of gross domestic product [GDP]) necessary to sustain them. Despite relatively high funding, most European countries introduced market-oriented reforms in the 1980s and 1990s (Saltman and Figueras 1998). Countries that have invested little in their health systems (less than 2 percent of GDP) have not been able to fully deliver health services through the public sector, even if the rhetoric of a universal public provider has continued.

In India, the state of Kerala proves that achieving good health outcomes, particularly low infant and child mortality rates, is possible even at India's levels of economic development. But even in Kerala, the vision of complete public provision is not a reality—health spending in both the public and private sectors is greater there than in other states. Whereas Kerala may have better public clinics than most states, 69 percent of outpatient clinical visits are in the private sector. The distribution of public spending in Kerala is remarkably equitable, but the result is due in part to the fact that many of the richer households in Kerala use only private hospitals. In Kerala, as elsewhere in India, the emergence of a two-track health care system is of growing concern (see chapter 7).

The experience of other states (such as Bihar and Uttar Pradesh) also reveals troubling realities that are not conducive to the rhetorical vision of a universal, vertically integrated, publicly provided system:

• India's state governments have not provided the funds necessary to make that vision a reality. In contrast to other countries that have had more success with public health systems, India's fiscal effort has been much smaller. As chapter 8 shows, India's public spending on health is among the lowest in the world, whereas its proportion of private spending on health is among the highest.

- The states have not demonstrated the capacity to provide curative health services of sufficiently high quality to attract users, despite lower direct costs to consumers. As shown in chapter 6, users prefer the private sector in its various forms for most curative care.

- In most states a strong pro-rich bias exists in the distribution of the benefits of public curative care. Chapter 7 shows that it is not uncommon to find a ratio of 3 rupees (Rs) spent on the richest 20 percent of the population for every Rs1 spent on the poorest 20 percent.

Endeavoring to correct present imbalances by allocating more public spending to the health sector has its own complexities. The political risk taking and bureaucratic commitment required to reallocate the funds from other uses has been too great to be attempted; any proposal for a significant expansion of the very low level of public spending on health would instead have to show how the additional spending would be financed. The mandatory purchase of

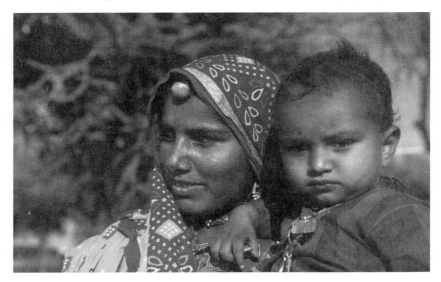

Mother and child (PHOTOGRAPH BY CURT CARNEMARK/THE WORLD BANK PHOTO LIBRARY)

insurance is one option, with the poor covered from public revenues; another option is the combination of mandated benefits and mandatory insurance. Some cost recovery could be accomplished at the point of service, but the level of recovery would be significant only where it is least important—in those ambulatory care goods and services for which private providers are the most viable.

These realities are not immutable, but one cannot simply assume that they will disappear. They can, however, be changed through institutional reforms and strong political commitment. Viable options for the health system must be technically feasible, consistent with public sector capacity, and capable of commanding sufficient social and political support to be sustainable.

Focusing on Four Critical Activities in the Health System

The focus in this report is on four critical sets of activities selected from within the larger set of functions of the health system:

a. Oversight of the health system

b. Delivery of public health services

c. Delivery of ambulatory curative services

d. Delivery and financing of inpatient care.

Other health care functions—human resource development, pharmaceuticals, technology development and assessment, and knowledge management—must also be improved, but this report does not concentrate on those functions. Options in those areas ought to support decisions made in the four critical areas of activity just listed.

The Approach to Reform

A number of pitfalls await health care reformers; among them are making ill-advised international comparisons, choosing a fixed model rather than clear goals that encourage experimentation, and striving for uniformity where variation is needed.

International Comparisons

International comparisons of health care systems, although useful, should be made with care (box 1.1). Debates about the latest policy changes in North America or Europe cannot directly inform the next steps for India, whose demographic and institutional realities are so different from those of high-income countries. Even if a health system with universal availability through a vertically integrated, public sector monopoly is the chosen vision—and whether such a vision is the right one is hardly clear—immediate expansion of the public sector is not likely to be the best way to implement it. Better understanding and use of current resources in the private sector as well as in the public sector would be a more realistic approach.

The Need for Experimentation

Because reforms need to emerge from continuing analysis, public discourse, and experimentation, this report does not propose a single vision for India's health sector. Indeed, any one of many different pathways could lead to improvements in health, in health-related financial security, and in the responsiveness of the health care system. More important than the attempt to define the best path in detail is the attempt to articulate the criteria that broadly define a better health system. A better health system would do the following:

- Keep people well informed about the choices that affect their health and health care

- Provide to everyone a minimum level of high-quality, high-impact health services—such as immunizations, safe-motherhood programs, communicable disease control, family planning, and first-referral clinical services

- Pool health funds to reduce the financial risk from catastrophic illness

Box 1.1 Lessons on Health Reform in Wealthy Countries

The health systems of many high-income countries have been reformed in the past few decades. The main motivation of such reforms has often been runaway costs, and the main challenge has been to control costs while maintaining or broadening access to high-quality care for all members of society. A number of the lessons learned are germane to the Indian agenda:

- Access and infrastructure are easier to expand than to cut back.
- The preferred strategy for controlling costs is to empower consumers and tie payments to services provided to patients within the context of an overall health budget.
- Reforms in one part of the health sector, such as insurance mechanisms for selected services or populations or subsidies for certain services or drugs, require careful monitoring of access to services and of expenditures in other parts of the health sector.
- The payment systems least successful in controlling costs or in promoting equity are those without a single payer or single set of rules, such as the fragmented fee-for-service systems in the United States and India.
- Carefully implemented strategies to provide insurance through full or partial risk sharing along with certain types of managed care have been best able to control costs without compromising quality and access.
- Payment mechanisms used in high-income countries require sophisticated information systems and administrative structures.

Source: OECD (1992, 1994).

• Maintain services at an affordable and socially sustainable level.

In identifying options for India's future health system, we look at the full set of tools available to government, including oversight functions, financing, managing nonfinancial inputs, and service delivery options (table 1.1).

The diversity of the Indian population and the large variations among the states are major themes of this report. We consider these differences with special concern for the most vulnerable segments of Indian society and with the understanding that recommendations for the whole of India or even for groups of states run the risk of oversimplification. Health is a shared responsibility of the central government and the states. The degree of discretion enjoyed by states in any aspect of health policy varies by state and by issue. In some public health activities, the central government will likely take the lead through centrally sponsored schemes; but for curative services, states already differ enormously in what they provide and in how well they provide it. Such differences, along with variations between the states in social expectations and in the political positions that leaders take, also affect the choices to be made at the state and national levels.

International experience tells us that there is no single correct way to shape a country's health system. Within India, priorities and options should vary according to the conditions prevailing in the various states and districts. If the country approaches the task of reforming its health care system in the collaborative, wide-ranging manner of these studies and with vigilance for the welfare of the weakest segments of society, the health system may well become able to continually evolve in a manner that is accountable, equitable, and affordable for all Indians.

Table 1.1 Examples of Health System Functions and Challenges in India

FUNCTION	EXAMPLES	CHALLENGES
Oversight		
Policy setting	• National Health Policy (Government 1983) • National Population Policy (MOHFW 2000b) • State health policy	• How can health needs and interventions be prioritized? • How can policy intentions be translated into decisions on allocation of resources? • How can the needs of vulnerable populations be addressed? • How can a meaningful framework for private sector participation in health be provided?
Regulation and setting standards	• Regulation of drug quality, private nursing homes • Promoting quality assurance systems (e.g., accreditation of hospitals, licensing of providers) • Health insurance regulation	• How can regulation be done positively to influence behavior of public and private providers? • How can sanctions be enforced effectively? • How can market failures of private health insurance be ameliorated?
Providing incentives	• Subsidizing health providers to work in remote areas • Duty exemptions, free land for hospitals • Providing materials, drugs, and training to providers to follow good clinical practices	• How can subsidies be structured so they can be monitored? • How can direct subsidies be directed toward public objectives?
Developing partnerships	• Developing networks of providers who offer good quality, who contribute to national programs • Training NGOs and for-profit providers in national guidelines. • Sharing information on disease surveillance	• How can providers who contribute to national objectives be distinguished from those who do not? • What are the mechanisms to develop meaningful partnerships?
Providing information and advocacy	• Disclosing good- and poor-quality health providers and products • Communicating standards for care and pricing to the public and to industry	• How can information to consumers, providers, financiers, and government be used to improve accountability, quality, use, and costs of health services? • Should government buy or directly produce its information services?

Monitoring and evaluation	• Measuring use of health services by identified groups (e.g., poor, women, SC/ST) • Measuring health outcomes • Monitoring efficiency of health services and programs	• How can the capacity to develop and monitor health system functions and outcomes be strengthened? • Who should conduct the monitoring and evaluation activities? • How can monitoring results be fed into planning and budgeting?
Financing		
Raising revenues	• User fees (out-of-pocket) • Tax revenue and user charges • Insurance premiums	• What is an adequate level of public funding? • How can private spending on heath be better collected and used?
Pooling resources	• Health insurance (private for-profit, nonprofit community financing, social insurance)	• What should be the level of prepayment? • What should be in the package of benefits and who will provide the services? • How will the risks be pooled? • How will the poor be subsidized?
Purchasing services	• Contracting for clinical and nonclinical services • Salaries and grants for public providers and institutions • Fee-for-service payments	• When and how should government contract for clinical and nonclinical services? • What is the best way to pay for publicly provided services? • Are there ways to move away from user fees (which raise health costs) and toward global budgets and capitation?
Managing nonfinancial inputs		
Providing drugs, health professionals, capital, etc.	• Producing drugs and vaccines • Training medical professionals • Developing health information systems • Building hospitals and clinics	• Should government produce or purchase these services? • Should government change the standards for these inputs (e.g., remove PHC inpatient beds) or the way it purchases them (e.g., rational drug procurement)? • What types of health professionals and skills are needed?

(Table continues on the following page.)

Table 1.1 (continued)

FUNCTION	EXAMPLES	CHALLENGES
Service provision		
Delivery of public health services	• Communicable disease control programs • Behavior change communications (e.g., AIDS prevention, family planning promotion)	• What is the best way to organize public programs? • How should programs be decentralized to states and districts? • How can programs be more equitable, efficient? • Should government buy or directly produce its information services?
Ambulatory clinical care	• Unqualified allopathic practitioners solo practice • Nonallopathic private practitioners • Private solo practitioners • Public subcenters, PHCs, hospital outpatient departments	• How should public provision of ambulatory curative care be continued? • Can private nonallopathic and unqualified allopathic be used to provide health services of public priority to extend coverage?
Inpatient care	• Private nursing homes • Trust hospitals • Public hospitals	• Should public hospitals be organized to be more efficient? • How can catastrophic costs of hospitalization be ameliorated?

Note: We do not explicitly outline demand function interventions. Interventions in information and advocacy, regulation, and standard setting are largely intended to influence demand and correct for market failures. MOHFW is Ministry of Health and Family Welfare; SC/ST is scheduled castes and tribes; PHC is primary health center.

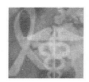

CHAPTER 2

Problems of the Public and Private Sectors

Before proceeding to policy options, we briefly sketch the structures and problems of the public and private health sectors in India. Existing research on Indian health care is at its weakest with regard to the private sector; this study is the first to synthesize the literature on that sector.

In broad terms, the public sector is vast, but it is sorely underfunded and not nearly large enough to meet the current health needs of the country. Moreover, it is overly centralized and rigid in its planning, politically manipulated, and poorly managed. The private sector is growing quickly but it is undirected and unregulated. It is without standards of care, is populated by many unqualified practitioners, and likely provides far too many inappropriate treatments. Whether seen in the public or private sector, patients finance much of their care out-of-pocket.

Current Structure of the Public Sector

The public sector has been organized largely to finance and deliver curative care, although it also implements a number of centrally sponsored programs for family welfare and disease control. These programs are almost exclusively delivered through an enormous array of underfunded public institutions.[1]

Internationally comparable data on manpower and facilities are weak, but what are available suggest that the number of medical personnel and hospital beds in India's public sector—although huge in absolute numbers—is, in per capita terms, well below the comparable ratios in other low-income countries. Combining the data for public and private sectors, the per capita number of physicians in India is about average for low-income countries, whereas the ratios for nurses and midwives and for hospital beds are well below average (table 2.1).[2] The rate of outpatient visits and hospitalizations are poor indicators of disease levels in a country, and differences in definitions and data collection methods between countries require that such data be treated with caution. The data do suggest, however, that hospital and outpatient utilization in India in the public and private sectors (total) is lower than in most countries, including low-income countries (table 2.2).

Under the Indian Constitution, the responsibility for public health is shared by the central, state, and local levels of government, but the delivery of public sector health services is effectively a state responsibility. State and local governments account for about three-fourths of public spending on health, but states vary widely in the size of their health budgets (see chapter 8). Decentralization of state authority also varies widely by state. At the local level, only large cities have a significant financial authority. In some states, however, local bodies have a significant responsibility for managing services and implementing national or state government programs.

Problems of the Public Sector

As documented in many previous studies, the delivery of health services in India's public sector is rife with problems (World Bank 1995, 1996, 1997b, 2000c; Mukhopadhyay 1997). High levels of poverty lead to, and are exacerbated by, poor health conditions, and poor governance creates a weak environment for reform. The public sector health system also suffers from poor management, low service quality, and weak finances. Weak management and the low quality

Table 2.1 International Comparisons of Health Care Work Force and Hospital Beds, 1990–98
(per 1,000 persons)

COUNTRY	PHYSICIANS	NURSES	MIDWIVES	HOSPITAL BEDS
India				
Public sector	0.2	—	0.2	0.4
Total	1.0	0.9	0.2	0.7
All countries, by income				
Low income	0.7	1.6	0.3	1.5
Middle income	1.8	1.9	0.6	4.3
High income	1.8	7.5	0.5	7.4
All	1.5	3.3	0.4	3.3

— Not available.
Note: Data are the most recent available in the time period. Income is unweighted per capita GNP in 1999 U.S. dollars: Low income, less than $755; middle income, $756–$9,265; high income, more than $9,265.
Source: World Development Indicators (World Bank 2000d), except for India: CBHI (various years) and MOHFW (2000a); and nurse and midwife data (WHO 1999).

Table 2.2 International Comparisons of Health Service Utilization and DALYs Lost, 1990–98

COUNTRY	INPATIENT ADMISSIONS PER CAPITA PER YEAR (PERCENT)	AVERAGE LENGTH OF INPATIENT STAY (DAYS)	OUTPATIENT VISITS (PER CAPITA PER YEAR)	DALYs LOST (PER 1,000 PERSONS PER YEAR)
India				
Public sector	0.7	14	0.7	—
Total	1.7	12	3.9[a]	274
All countries, by income				
Low income	5	13	3	256[b]
Middle income	10	11	5	256[b]
High income	15	16	8	119
All	9	13	6	234

— Not available.
Note: Data are the most recent available in the time period. DALYs, disability-adjusted life years. Income is unweighted per capita GNP in 1999 U.S. dollars: Low income, less than $755; middle income, $756–$9,265; high income, more than $9,265.
a. Includes all visits to health providers, regardless of system of medicine.
b. Estimated for low-income and middle-income countries combined.
Source: World Development Indicators (World Bank 2000d), except for India utilization data (National Sample Survey Organisation 1998) and DALYs (WHO 1999).

of services are related problems that include structural and institutional issues as well as constraints on processes and skills.

Public health management in India suffers from overly centralized and inflexible planning and control of resources; high levels of political interference in staff postings and transfers in some of the larger states; a failure to integrate programs devoted to family welfare, nutrition, and disease control and different levels of care; and the neglect of approaches that would encourage the private sector to meet public policy objectives.

An example of inflexible planning is that staffing norms for auxiliary nurse midwives are based on a standard population coverage, although birthrates vary widely across the country. As a result, the workload to deliver immunizations to children in high-fertility states like Uttar Pradesh and Bihar is more than double that in a low-fertility state like Tamil Nadu (Satia 1999).

Managers have neither the authority nor the information necessary for accountable decisionmaking. Human resource systems offer little by way of monitoring, staff incentives, or in-service training, and the result is an undisciplined, poorly performing staff. An inappropriate mix of skills is one of the most critical issues, as large numbers of key posts remain vacant, particularly in rural areas. According to the established staffing norms for existing subcenters, primary health centers, and community health centers, the shortfalls range from 17 percent for auxiliary nurse midwives, to 28 percent for doctors, to 47 percent for male multipurpose workers and nurse midwives (Ministry of Health and Family Welfare 2000a).

The problems are not simply that the staff norms are too ambitious, that the selection of staff is inappropriate, and that too few health workers are being trained. The problems extend to insufficient pay in the public sector, particularly in comparison with the private sector, unsatisfactory living conditions in rural areas, and limited professional opportunities. However, questions of staff motivation and incentives have not been well studied in the health sector and need a more systematic assessment (chapter 5).

The quality of health services is not well monitored in either the public or private sectors because meaningful standards and quality

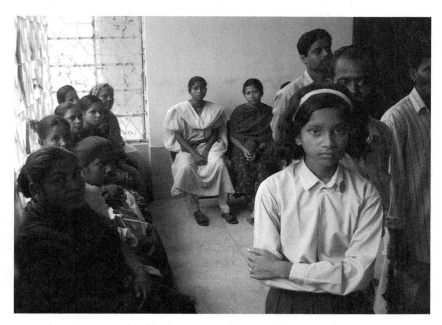

Patiently waiting at a health clinic (PHOTOGRAPH BY GEETANJALI CHOPRA/HEMANT MEHTA/ THE WORLD BANK)

assurance systems are absent. Hence, little is known about clinical outcomes, clinical quality, management quality, or quality from the perspective of the user. Public sector health services are largely underutilized in rural areas—according to STEM (2000), bed occupancy rates of rural inpatient facilities in Uttar Pradesh are around 30 percent—and one reason is the perceived poor quality of service.

The public sector is further constrained by staffing limitations, particularly in poor and remote areas that are also not served by the formal private sector, and is more hampered by weaknesses in supervision, maintenance, drugs, and supplies.

Despite the establishment of a large public network of health providers, public spending on health has stagnated at levels of around 1 percent of GDP, far below what is needed to provide basic health care to the population (World Bank 1997b; Mahal, Srivastava, and Sanan 2001). The bulk of public spending on primary health care has been spread too thinly to be effective, while the referral linkages to secondary care have also suffered (Tulasidhar 1996; Mukhopadhyay 1997). As in other countries, preventive and promotive health services take a back seat to curative care. Yet preventive care is almost exclusively provided through the public sector: an estimated 90 percent of immunizations and 60 percent of prenatal care is provided through the public sector (IIPS 2000; Background Paper 18). The states, which bear between 75 percent and 90 percent of the burden of public health spending, have their funds largely tied up in "nonplan" salary expenditures (Duggal 1997; Reddy and Selvaraju 1994). The disparity between rich and poor states is apparently increasing, while expenditures are not reaching the implementing bodies, particularly the more geographically remote ones (Rao, Ramana, and Murthy 1997).

Structure of the Private Sector

In India, the private health sector is commonly understood to refer to private, for-profit, medically trained providers. Their range of practice varies from solo practices and small nursing homes (inpatient facilities with usually less than 30 beds) to large corporate hospitals. However, the set of nongovernment actors involved is much broader and includes nonprofit entities and providers of Indian systems of medicine such as auyervedic and unani. Many untrained providers offer a combination of systems of medicine, although Western medicine (allopathy) tends to dominate. The private sector also offers ancillary services such as diagnostic centers, ambulance services, and pharmacies. In addition, a large number of private actors provide services or manage other inputs to the sector (construction companies, consultancy firms). A few private companies and community organizations finance health services for their members, but overall the private sector's formal role in health financing has been limited.

The number of studies concerning the private health sector has increased in recent years, but the present work is the first to attempt a systematic synthesis of the literature on the private health sector. Three Indian institutions have created a single database on private health sector studies in India; the studies point toward the rapid growth of private sector health provision, particularly by for-profit and nonqualified providers.[3] Despite this growth, relatively few studies have been conducted on the for-profit private sector in India. Studies on the nonprofit sector tend to have small coverage, and many have weak methodologies. Also, some key innovations that have been taking place in India in the last few years lack documentation; these innovations have been in areas such as the contracting of services in the public sector; partnerships between public and private sectors; payment systems; and the use of subsidies.

The data on health financing, also limited, suggest that, throughout the country, health financing is predominantly private and paid out-of-pocket from individual consumers in a fragmentary way to many different types of service providers. The lack of a clear health policy framework and inadequate implementation mechanisms at national, state, and local levels toward private sector health are cited in Background Papers 6–8 as major reasons why the research and information base for planning and evaluation of the private sector in India is very limited.

Although the most recent data are quite weak, they suggest that the private provision of health is growing rapidly and is the major source of outpatient and inpatient health care across India. At the time of Independence (1947), the private sector involved in allopathic medicine was quite small. Only about 8 percent of all medical institutions in the provinces were operated by private agencies, and another 5 percent in the nongovernment sector were receiving government grants-in-aid (Bhore, Amesur, and Banerjee 1946). By 1995, government publications estimate that private hospitals represented more than two-thirds of all hospitals and nearly 40 percent of the hospital beds (see table 2.3). However, a census of private facilities undertaken in Andhra Pradesh in 1993 found that the actual number of hospitals was 3.8 times larger than the official number, and the actual number of hospital beds was 10.5 times larger. In more recent estimates, private hospitals represent 93 percent of all hospitals and 64 percent of all hospital beds nationwide. In addition to these allo-

Table 2.3 Health Care Work Force and Health Facilities in the Public and Private Sectors in India, Selected Years, 1981–98

INDICATOR AND MEASURE	VALUE
Doctors	
Total number (1998) (includes all systems) (CBHI)	1,109,853
Population per doctor	880
Percentage of doctors in rural areas (1981) (census)	41
Percentage of all doctors in private sector (estimated)	80–85
Nurses	
Total number (1996)	867,184
Population per nurse	976
Doctors per nurse (1996)	1.4
Hospitals	
Total number (1996)	15,097
Population per hospital	56,058
Percentage of hospitals in private sector	68
Estimated total number of hospitals	71,860
Estimated population per hospital	11,744
Estimated percentage of hospitals in private sector	93
Hospital Beds	
Total number (1996) (CBHI)	623,819
Population per hospital bed	1,357
Percentage of beds in rural areas	21
Percentage of beds in private sector	37
Estimated total number of beds	1,217,427
Estimated population per bed	693
Percentage of beds in private sector	64
PHCs	
Total number	22,975
Rural population per PHC	27,364

Note: PHCs, primary health centers. The estimate for manpower is based on medical council lists. The estimate for the number of hospitals and beds are based on the extent of underestimation in government (Central Bureau of Health Intelligence [CBHI]) data found in Andhra Pradesh in a 1993 census of all hospitals by the Director of Health Services and the Andhra Pradesh Vaidya Vidhan Parishad; they found 2,802 hospitals and 42,192 hospital beds in the private sector in Andhra Pradesh as against only 266 hospitals and 11,103 beds officially reported by the CBHI in that year. Thus, compared with the official (CBHI) data, the number of private hospitals was larger by a factor of 10.5, and the number of beds by a factor of 3.8.
Source: Estimates are by Duggal (2000) and Nandraj (Background Paper 6). Background Paper 6 drew on CBHI (various years), Census Commissioner of India (1981), and Ministry of Health and Family Welfare (2000a).

pathic facilities, an estimated 2,800 hospitals (and 46,000 hospital beds) are operating under the Indian systems of medicine, the vast majority of which are in the private sector.

Data on the health workforce in the private sector are hard to come by. Between 400,000 and 470,000 allopathic doctors were estimated to have been in practice in 1997 (Planning Commission 1998), with about 80–85 percent of them in the private sector (Duggal 2000). However, many doctors employed in the public sector also work in the private sector, with one study in Delhi showing 85 percent of public sector doctors also practicing in the private sector (Chawla 2000). Of the 120,000 doctors estimated to have been practicing Indian systems of medicine in 1981, about 85 percent were in the private sector. Although information on the numbers of private doctors is limited, estimates about the numbers of other medical and paramedical professions in the private sector are not available.

Estimating the number of informal providers is even more problematic, since they are not registered, and many work part-time. Conservative estimates put the number of nonqualified rural medical practitioners at 1.25 million; almost all are solo practitioners located in outpatient settings (Rohde and Viswanathan 1995). A census in three districts in Andhra Pradesh found about one non-MBBS (Bachelor of Medicine and Bachelor of Surgery) doctor per 2,000 population (Rao, Ramana, and Murthy 1997), which would extrapolate to about 500,000 nonqualified medical practitioners. A number of other studies have examined the role of traditional practitioners in its various dimensions (BAIF 1997; Kumar and Patel 1992; Chand 1988; Yesudian 1994). Broadly, these studies reveal that the majority of qualified solo practitioners practice in urban areas. Untrained practitioners, faith healers, traditional birth attendants, priests, and local medicine women and men largely cater to the rural areas. In rural as well as urban areas, however, the allopathic treatment is the dominant type of care provided.

Population surveys on the use of health services indicate an increasing use of health services through the private sector. Between the 42nd Round of the National Sample Survey in 1986–87 and the 52nd

Round in 1995–96 (NSSO 1992, 1998), the proportion of people using care outside the public sector increased (table 2.4). The vast majority of people both in urban and in rural areas (more than 80 percent) use the private sector for outpatient curative services as a first line of treatment. As already mentioned, the qualifications of practitioners and the systems of medicine used for outpatient care vary widely. Indigenous and folk practitioners, along with traditional providers, are particularly used as a first line of outpatient treatment in rural areas (Rohde and Viswanathan 1995). For inpatient care, the majority of people are now using the private sector for hospitalization. States differ a great deal in the extent to which their populations use private services as well as in the level of poverty and type of service provided.

The majority of private hospitals are small (less than 30 beds); they are usually each owned by one person, a practicing doctor. Although some private hospitals are well known, very few of the private hospitals or private hospital beds are in the tertiary sector, comprising roughly 1 percent of the total number of institutions, whereas charitable hospitals cater to about 4 percent of hospitalized patients (NSSO 1998). Although partnerships own a number of hospitals, relatively few are corporate, public limited, or trust hospitals. Most of the nursing homes are owned by a doctor entrepreneur and

Table 2.4 Distribution of Outpatient and Inpatient Health Services across the Public and Private Sectors in India, 1986–87 and 1995–96
(percent)

| | 1986–87 | | 1995–96 | |
TREATMENT OF AILING PERSONS	RURAL	URBAN	RURAL	URBAN
Not treated	18	11	17	9
Treated as outpatients				
Public	26	28	19	20
Private	74	72	81	80
Treated as inpatients				
Public	60	60	44	43
Private	40	40	56	57

Source: National Sample Survey Organisation (1992, 1998).

provide general curative medical and maternity services. The large private hospitals are either owned by trusts or are corporate enterprises and offer more specialized services.

In the typical staffing pattern, small hospitals have fewer than four physicians working at the hospital and depend on visiting consultants. For example, in Muraleedharan's study of private hospitals in Chennai (1999b), the consultant physician averaged just over three hours per day in a hospital and visited at least two different practice localities. Muraleedharan also found that about two-thirds of private hospitals had on average about two government doctors on their panels of consultants, averaging about two government doctors per private hospital. The presence of government doctors in private hospitals has been reported in other parts of the country as well, even in states where private practice by government doctors is prohibited.

Problems with the Private Sector

One of the main problems with the private health sector is that it has grown in an undirected fashion, with virtually no effective guidance on the location and scope of practice, and without effective standards for quality of care or public disclosure on practices and pricing. Quality of health care in the private sector has become a major concern in the popular press. But few reports systematically examine the quality provided in the private sector; hence, generalizations about the care provided by such a large and heterogeneous private sector are difficult to make.

The available studies are quite limited in scope. For example, a study in two districts of Maharashtra found a large number of practitioners practicing modern medicine without being qualified to do so. It also found several hospitals that were operating without any licenses or registration and did not have even the basic infrastructure and personnel to carry out their functions (Nandraj and Duggal 1996). More-recent studies of private medical hospitals in Calcutta and Bombay also indicate that private sector facilities are in poor condition and are frequently used to perform medically unnecessary procedures (Nandraj, Khot, and Menon 1999).

Studies that have examined provider behavior with respect to specific diseases, such as tuberculosis and diarrhea, have documented significant deficiencies among both qualified and untrained practitioners (Balambal, Faggarajamma, and Rahman 1997; Bhandari 1992; Uplekar and Shepard 1991). Whether clinical management is better in the public sector is not clear, as these studies tend to compare private sector treatment behavior with standard treatment protocols and not with how patients are actually treated in the public sector.

Data on the performance of private hospitals are especially difficult to obtain. Most hospitals, including many of the large hospitals, do not have patient records or information systems to report on performance. Of the studies that have examined work volume, Homan and Thankappan's study in Kerala (1999) showed that private city hospitals had higher occupancy rates than public hospitals. The available evidence also suggests that private hospitals provide more intensive and expensive services, using more x-rays and laboratory tests per patient than the public sector (Homan and Thankappan 1999). This finding may suggest good care or unnecessary expense; nonetheless, simple diagnostic tests such as x-rays and laboratory tests have been shown to be vastly underused in the public sector (World Bank 1997b).

Other evidence of overutilization of procedures and diagnostic services in the private sector more clearly accounts for an increase in health care expenditures in the private sector (see box 2.1). An example is the very high rates of cesarean deliveries in a number of communities, often more than 40 percent (Pai and others 1999; Muraleedharan 1997; Kannan and others 1991). Although the appropriate proportion of deliveries that should be done by cesarean section is widely debated, the rates found in India are far beyond what could be considered acceptable (WHO 1985). In numerous countries, the influence of the private sector as well as fee-for-service payments to doctors has been shown to be associated with increased rates of

Box 2.1 A Proactive Public Health Provider

Shyam is a Harijan, a member of the scheduled caste, living in southern Uttar Pradesh. When his 5-year-old son fell ill with vomiting and diarrhea, Shyam took him to an unqualified private practitioner in the nearest town. Shyam did not consult the nearby (public sector) primary health center, as he had heard from neighbors that it had no medicines.

The boy received injections and medicines of substances unknown to his illiterate parents, but he failed to improve. He was then taken to a private nursing home, where he was admitted and given an intravenous solution (locally known as "bottles") for two days. The child recovered, but the total cost of his treatment was Rs 500.

Meanwhile, the child's 12-year-old brother had developed the same symptoms. This time the family consulted the government hospital. One of the health workers at the government hospital took the child to his residential private practice, where he gave two bottles for Rs 200 and medicines from the market, which cost another Rs 300.

Very soon the third son, aged 14, also developed diarrhea and vomiting. All three children eventually recovered, but the family had spent more than Rs 1,500 on their children's medical expenses. All of the money was borrowed from neighbors and Shyam's employer.

The Medical Officer in charge of Shyam's primary health center heard about the case and visited the village to investigate the outbreak. He took samples from the family's source of drinking water—an open water tank—and had them tested at a government laboratory. The tests showed bacterial contamination. The Medical Officer returned to the village to treat the water and counsel the villagers on the importance of boiling or treating potentially contaminated water.

Source: World Bank (2000a).

cesarean sections (Cai and others 1998; Stafford 1990; De Regt and others 1986). Similar detrimental effects on medical practice arise from the marketing practices of the pharmaceutical industry. A number of studies in India have pointed to medically inappropriate treatment by private providers who are linked to incentives provided by pharmaceutical companies and salesmen to increase sales of their products (Shah 1996; Thaver and others 1998; Phadke 1998; Greenhalgh 1986). In this report, we build on these findings and examine in more detail how the private sector functions.

Notes

1. As of 1999, the public infrastructure included about 137,000 subcenters, 28,000 dispensaries, 23,000 primary health centers (PHCs), 3,500 urban family welfare facilities, 3,000 community health centers (CHCs, which are 30-bed secondary hospitals), and an additional 12,000 secondary and tertiary hospitals. In rural areas, the public sector work force in 1999 included 29,000 doctors, 18,000 nurse midwives, 134,000 auxiliary nurse midwives, 73,000 male multipurpose workers, 21,000 pharmacists, and 60,000 paramedics plus nontechnical workers (Ministry of Health and Family Welfare 2000a). Data on the size of the public sector workforce in urban areas are not available.

2. The number of hospital beds in the private sector in India is likely more than double the number recorded in government estimates, so the public-private total for India is therefore about 1 bed, instead of 0.7 bed, per 1,000 population and thus about two-thirds, instead of one-half, of the average number for low-income countries.

3. Background Papers 6–8, published together as "Private Health Sector in India: Review and Annotated Bibliography," are available electronically at the following address: http://wbln0018.worldbank.org/SAR/India/HealthESW/AR/cover.nsf/HomePage/1?OpenDocument.

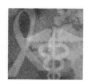

CHAPTER 3

Policy Actions for Critical Health System Activities

This chapter outlines several feasible public actions (table 3.1) for improving the four critical health system activities—oversight of the health sector, public health services, ambulatory care, and inpatient care and financing. For each activity, we present the justification for public intervention. We also present the broad advantages and disadvantages ("pros" and "cons") of each proposed action. Because of the variation in state conditions, not all options will have the same relevance or attraction to the different states. In chapter 4, we will examine how to put some of these options together, by assessing which actions are more important for states under different conditions and by examining programs that cut across the main activities discussed in this chapter.

We provide our judgments of the possible pros and cons of each action as an aid to citizens, planners, and policymakers in addressing change. Some caveats are in order: The list of advantages and disadvantages is of course not comprehensive; others might be realized instead. Moreover, advantages realized may not turn out to have been sufficient to justify the action, and disadvantages realized may be manageable.

Our basic approach is to examine options for change, not for maintaining the status quo. Maintaining the health system in its present form will become untenable in India. The health transition is polarizing health conditions while bringing higher health care

Table 3.1 Summary of Actions for Critical Areas of Activity in the Health System

AREA OF ACTIVITY	ACTION
Health system oversight	1. Develop partnerships with private sector to share information, improve quality, cooperate on service provision 2. Support independent organizations to measure performance in public and private sectors 3. Facilitate health-advocacy organizations that are independent both of public providers and private associations to work as consumer advocates 4. Support professional self-regulation 5. Strengthen formal regulation of health inputs (drug quality) 6. Formalize public sector regulation of private providers

Public health service delivery	1. Concentrate efforts on programs for the "unfinished agenda" by:
	    a. Increasing funding
	    and
	    b. Increasing effectiveness
	2. Initiate and strengthen programs in noncommunicable diseases in states well advanced in the epidemiological transition
	3. Reduce centrally sponsored schemes, turn over the resources to the states, reassign functions of central Ministry of Health and Family Welfare
	4. Reinvest heavily in public health systems generally

Ambulatory curative services	1. Focus public resources strategically by:
	    a. Revitalizing the network of public facilities in disadvantaged areas
	    and
	    b. Purchasing curative care from the private sector when possible, limiting public provision from primary health centers (PHCs) and subcenters in those areas
	2. Expand ambulatory curative care coverage for the poor through the use of demand-side mechanisms that give the poorest access to publicly subsidized discounts at either public or certified private providers
	or
	3. Revitalize the entire network of public sector facilities to raise quality of publicly provided services

Inpatient care and health insurance	1. Encourage multiple insurance pools with strong regulation, using employer or union schemes, community financing, and public insurance *or* 2. Initiate compulsory purchase of "single payer" insurance coverage *or* 3. Rely on the introduction of private voluntary health insurance 4. Invest in quality of care, especially in public sector secondary hospitals serving rural areas, but increase cost recovery with or without prepayment mechanisms to improve equality 5. Make public hospitals autonomous, and fund their services publicly

costs, new technologies, and rising expectations. Under such conditions, low levels of public investment in health, overly centralized planning, inefficient public services, heavy reliance on private, out-of-pocket financing, little public oversight of the expanding private sector, and a loosely regulated health insurance market are not likely to be sustained. The demand for change is increasing, not diminishing. The question is whether the changes will involve tinkering at the margins or more substantial reforms; stopgap reactions or planned, publicly considered improvements.

Health System Oversight

Rationale for Public Sector Intervention

Oversight, a key function of the health system, affects all other activities. As a clear "public good" that benefits all individuals, oversight is an area that requires public action. But, as Amartya Sen has repeatedly emphasized, public action is not synonymous with government action (Dreze and Sen 1995). In its half-century of Independence, India's experience with the "inspectorate raj" demonstrates the folly of assuming that creating a new government body with oversight powers and responsibilities will improve matters.

At its best, public oversight means empowering the people who use the health system. The goal is not to increase just the quality of services but also the accountability of the system. Health care is a complex and technical field, and health care providers will always have some information that their clients do not. Although empowerment does not mean learning to practice medicine, it does mean learning and having options. Any reforms will be far more effective in curtailing low-quality, fraudulent, and extortionist behaviors if people have the information, tools, and options they need to make better health choices.

Current and Emerging Policy Challenges

The private sector is a major provider of curative health services, both ambulatory and inpatient. The most plausible future for the health care system in India is that it will continue to be a mixed system of public and private institutions. Given that scenario, this study highlights a number of key policy challenges in the area of oversight (chapters that address them in more detail are in parentheses):

- What formal and informal steps can government take to improve performance of the private sector? Can government create a positive environment for the private sector as opposed to merely creating an inspectorate raj? (chapter 6)

- Can the quality and efficacy of health services be improved by increasing accountability for quality in both the private and the public sector? (chapter 7)

- Can the performance of the public sector be improved? Can the respective roles and resources of the center and the states be redistributed? Are there ways of organizing public sector services to be more efficient, equitable, and accountable? (chapter 7)

- Can consumer rights be promoted in ways that will boost public awareness of health and establish mechanisms for increasing the voice of the poor? (chapter 9)

- Can new and more responsive mechanisms be put in place to protect consumer interests and increase the social accountability of the health system? (chapter 9)

Actions for Improving Oversight

One of the most important considerations for government is whether it will spend more on overseeing the health sector, perhaps at the expense of public sector service delivery. One of the main gaps in India's health system, one that will not be closed by the private sector, is oversight. In particular, activities that will increase the measurability of health care providers and other actors in the health sector are sorely needed. These activities involve collecting and analyzing information on price, type, and volume of cases, and on service-quality indicators, including use of technology and clinical outcomes. It is also critical that such information be made available to the public and other providers.

Measurement is a prerequisite for greater public accountability, wider use of health insurance, and the strategic purchasing of health services. The potential benefits thus include more efficient health services and greater public accountability. One of the main difficulties in moving to a more measurable system is the uneven availability of technical expertise. Among the main problems to be managed in a more measurable health system are the risk of conflict with providers and the risk of manipulation of results. The remainder of this section considers various actions for improving oversight, with an emphasis on actions that improve measurability and accountability (table 3.1).

Action 1: Develop partnerships with the private sector to build networks of private and public providers; to seek cooperation on information, materials, training; and to use tools such as subsidies and contracting. This action covers a wide range of options for dealing with the private sector (figure 3.1), and much international experience is available on how well the partnerships work (table 3.2).

- *Pro.* These options offer the possibility of improving efficiency and increasing service coverage at relatively low cost and without adding staff to the government. Contracting offers the prospect of increasing accountability while creating efficiencies that could not be attained with direct government provision of services.

- *Con.* As long as services are difficult to measure and social mandates and other expectations are unclear, the ability to contract effectively and to use subsidies is limited. Monitoring contracts requires expertise, the availability of which has not been well tested. Without goodwill from the public and private sectors, partnerships would not work well under existing circumstances. Another consideration is that many private providers from both for-profit and nongovernmental organizations (NGOs) do not work together except in their capacity as visiting consultants.

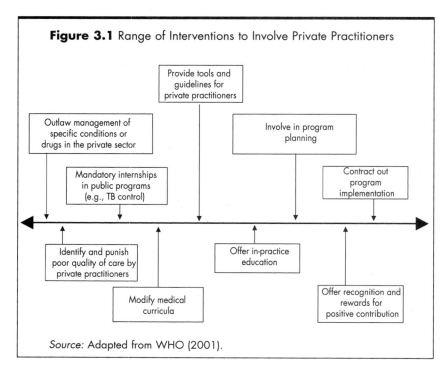

Figure 3.1 Range of Interventions to Involve Private Practitioners

Provide tools and guidelines for private practitioners

Outlaw management of specific conditions or drugs in the private sector

Involve in program planning

Mandatory internships in public programs (e.g., TB control)

Contract out program implementation

Identify and punish poor quality of care by private practitioners

Offer in-practice education

Modify medical curricula

Offer recognition and rewards for positive contribution

Source: Adapted from WHO (2001).

Bringing groups of providers together into networks for patient referral and the sharing of clinical responsibilities and information could create conflicts that might make some partnerships unworkable.

Action 2: Support independent organizations to measure performance among public and private providers.

- *Pro.* Such organizations would be honest brokers and best able to resist unwanted pressures from the public and private sectors. The broker might also be more efficient.

- *Con.* Maintaining independence would be difficult, and staff members could be confronted by personal threats.

Action 3: Facilitate the creation of "health advocacy" organizations independent of both public providers and private associations that would work

Table 3.2 International Examples of Varying Public-Private Mixes in the Delivery of Tuberculosis Care

STRATEGY AND INTERVENTION	EXAMPLE	EXPERIENCE
Public system *(excludes private providers)* Restrict antituberculosis drug sales	Chile Oman	Successful Successful
Mandate referrals	Syrian Arab Republic	To be evaluated
Parallel system *(independent public and private* *delivery systems)* Ignore	Many countries	Unsatisfactory
Compete for and attract tuber- culosis cases	Morocco, Peru	Successful
Collaborative system *(includes private providers)* Educate, inform providers	Many countries (long-term aim)	To be evaluated
Collaborate in delivery 1. Public health support services to private providers	Netherlands Jamnagar (India)	Successful To be evaluated
2. Incentives to individual providers for performance of specific tasks	China	Successful

3. Private agencies responsible
   for delivery of care to defined
   populations
	Chennai (India)
	Hyderabad (India)
	Bangladesh
	Manila
	Haiti
		Successful
		Successful
		Promising
		Promising
		To be evaluated

Source: WHO (2001).

as consumer advocates. This action would involve stimulating new organizations to become active representatives of people's concerns in the health sector.

- *Pro.* Such organizations hold the promise of greater participation by people in their health services and could help raise accountability and performance of health services at relatively low costs.

- *Con.* Few organizations currently have the capacity to advocate effectively, so that considerable time and effort would be needed to develop them. Preventing health advocacy groups from becoming "captured interests" of government or other political groups might also prove difficult. Consumer groups would tend to represent the middle class and elites before taking on the interests of the poor.

Action 4: Support professional self-regulation. This action would involve professional bodies in more active self-regulation through measures such as continuing medical education, accreditation of providers and facilities, or providing means for redress of patient complaints (box 3.1).

Box 3.1 A Quality Assurance Initiative in Mumbai

A Health Care Accreditation Council was recently formed in Mumbai[1] to help set quality standards for health care facilities. Uniquely, the council includes a range of stakeholders—representatives of private hospital owners, professional bodies, consumer organizations, and NGOs.

The council is being registered as a nonprofit body, with the initial funds for establishing the body raised from the founding members. The council is pursuing methods of financing for its continued work. Earlier attempts at setting up accreditation bodies for private sector health facilities have been unsuccessful, as they did not adequately involve key stakeholders. This initiative is an attempt to create a more positive environment for the private sector by involving it more meaningfully with other stakeholders in a quality assurance mechanism.

The council is focusing on small private hospitals, developing standards that will cover structural design, equipment, essential drugs, maintenance of medical records, and waste management. It is also addressing methods of rating facilities and how frequently to assess them. The council plans to develop standards for other health facilities in the near future.

- *Pro.* Self-regulation is likely to be more attractive to service providers than is regulation by the public sector.

- *Con.* The professional associations have done little self-regulation in the past and might not have the confidence of consumers or government, who might see these bodies as representing their own interests. Their technical capacity for self-regulation is untested.

Action 5: Strengthen formal public sector regulation of health factor inputs. The inputs include factors such as drug quality control. Such regulatory organizations exist in India, but they are underfinanced, poorly organized, and poorly functioning (box 3.2).

Box 3.2 Oversight Constraints and Opportunities: Reform of the Drug Control System in Uttar Pradesh

Drug control in Uttar Pradesh and many other states is generally known to be seriously defective. Substandard and fake drugs are on the market, and manufacturing and retailing establishments have poor standards. The harm from such a chaotic system can be as subtle as prolonged illness, medical complications, and higher rates of hospitalization, or they can be as dramatic as the 1974 Kanpur glucose scandal, in which contaminated glucose solution caused serious illness and death.

The reasons for the problem are numerous: a fragmented drug control organization with weak management, insufficient funds and material resources, poorly trained inspectors, inadequate sampling and laboratory capacity, and a reporting system that almost encourages corruption. By law, manufacturers and retailers should be inspected twice yearly, but many pharmacies have not seen an inspector for 10 years. Currently, reports on manufacturers rarely go to the Drug Control Authority; manufacturers need deal only with local officials in their effort to continue the production of substandard or spurious drugs.

Box 3.2 (continued)

More than 50 stakeholders of the drug control system (manufacturers, pharmacists, doctors, government administrators, NGOs, and political organizations) were interviewed about a reform program for the drug control system. The program would include establishment of a Drug Control Administration that would be independent of the Department of Health and have strengthened testing and inspection capabilities. More than 90 percent of those interviewed were in favor of reforms, but 80 percent also felt that they did not have the power to effect such reforms and that spurious drug manufacturers and corrupt traders and officials would continue to pose major problems. About 43 percent felt that corruption was widespread in the government bureaucracy, and 38 percent felt that corruption was widespread among drug manufacturers and wholesalers.

The government of Uttar Pradesh is now testing reforms of its drug control system. The reforms include instituting a direct state-level authority over inspections and supervision, with instantaneous, transparent computerized reporting. At the same time, the government is pursuing an expansion of its laboratories to test drug quality along with the option of using accredited private laboratories. The scheme would be financed out of modest fees charged to industry—fees that are expected to be lower than the bribes currently paid.

Sources: Dukes (2000); Basu (2000).

- *Pro.* Tackles important areas, such as pharmaceuticals, where low quality can place many Indians at risk. Input markets are more measurable than provider behaviors and hence easier to regulate.

- *Con.* The capacity of most states to regulate is quite weak, so that there is a substantial risk of not being able to enforce regulations, particularly as more costs are involved. Dealing with wealthy industries adds significant potential for corruption.

Action 6: Establish formal public sector regulation of private providers through legislation and legal enforcement. The private sector has many highly qualified and dedicated professionals but also many unqualified practitioners who pose a danger to public health.[2] One approach to reform would be to create a government agency responsible for the regulation of health care providers. The agency would set standards for, license, and receive complaints against providers; it would also inspect premises and otherwise generally take responsibility for bringing the private sector under public sector control.

- *Pro.* The current practice of responding only to complaints is a weak mechanism for disciplining abuses, especially given the overall weakness and slow pace of resolution of legal disputes.

- *Con.* First, in most states the capacity for regulation is quite weak. Second, to a large extent the expansion of the private sector has been facilitated by the general public's dissatisfaction with the quality of services in the public sector; proponents of regulation would thus have to explain why the public sector would nevertheless have the capacity to regulate the private sector. Third, formal regulation would run the risk of recreating an inspectorate raj in the health sector. As a result of the adversarial relationship thus created, more providers might be pushed outside the formal system of provision and regulation. Finally, experience in many other countries and with other activities demonstrates the risk of "regulatory capture," in which government regulators would form a coalition with existing providers to limit new entrants into the industry and use quality standards as a mechanism to limit competition and raise prices.

Public Health Service Delivery

Rationale for Public Sector Intervention

The rationale for public sector intervention in the delivery of public health services is strong. By definition, these services are organized in the public interest and take on issues of national concern such as family planning and HIV prevention. They address health problems with large externalities, particularly in communicable disease control, immunization, and safe motherhood.

Current and Emerging Policy Challenges

Some of the main challenges facing the delivery of public health services are expressed in the following questions.

- How can India best fight the HIV/AIDS epidemic, which has the real potential to undermine the health and development gains India has made since its Independence? (chapter 1)

- How can critical gaps be removed in planning, implementation, monitoring, technical leadership, and public communications? (chapter 7)

- When and how should effective programs be developed to address emerging public health priorities, such as the health consequences of smoking, mental illness, and injuries? (chapter 7)

- How can programs for existing public health priorities be strengthened while responsibilities and resources are decentralized to the states? (chapter 7)

Actions for Improving Public Health Services

Action 1: Concentrate effort on programs to address the "unfinished agenda." This action would entail increasing the funding for, and effectiveness of, programs to combat the conditions of the unfinished agenda, namely, the diseases of childhood and maternity, malnutrition, tuberculosis, and malaria. There is no single way to improve effectiveness, but the steps needed include increasing supervision and monitoring, invoking greater public involvement to increase accountability, enhancing communications strategies, and strengthening logistics systems and training. General efforts to improve public health capacity (action 4), greater decentralization of centrally sponsored schemes in some states (action 3) or greater partnerships with the private sector would also improve effectiveness.

- *Pro*. The conditions of the unfinished agenda still cause the largest burden of disease in India, particularly among the poor and in the states and districts with high mortality. Highly effective and inexpensive technologies exist to combat many of these conditions (box 3.3), and programs already exist to combat these conditions—they needn't be invented, just improved.

Box 3.3 Effective Technologies to Combat Communicable Diseases

The following drugs and technologies are highly effective when used correctly:
- Antibiotics for treating pneumonia are 90 percent effective. Cost: Rs 15 per course
- Oral rehydration for treating dehydration due to diarrhea is highly effective. Cost: Rs 20 per dose
- Measles vaccine is 85 percent effective in preventing measles. Cost: Rs 12 per vaccination
- Tuberculosis medicines are 95 percent effective in curing TB. Cost: Less than Rs 500 for a six-month course
- Antimalarials are 95 percent effective. Cost: Rs 6 per course
- Bednets, by reducing mosquito-borne malaria, can reduce child deaths by 25 percent. Cost: Rs 200 each

Plus:
- Latex condoms are highly effective at preventing HIV. Cost: Rs 650 for a year's supply

Source: WHO (2000a).

- *Con.* These programs need more than money and improvements to be effective—they need to be reorganized. Although cost-effective technologies exist, money spent on them will be wasted without a rise in political commitment, a more functional underlying delivery system, better management, and a greater capacity to innovate locally and develop partnerships across public and private sectors. This is more true among those states with weak capacity, where the need is greatest. Existing programs would also need to fill gaps in their design, such as targeting better nutrition during the weaning period and focusing on neonatal health care, which may be difficult to achieve.

Action 2: Initiate and strengthen programs addressing injuries and noncommunicable diseases in states well advanced in the epidemiological transition. The large and growing burden of disease requires the acceleration of preventive interventions against cardiovascular and tobacco-related illnesses, along with more comprehensive programs to prevent mental illness and injury.

- *Pro.* Noncommunicable diseases and injuries are already a major and growing part of India's disease burden, yet public health interventions to deal with them are still in their infancy. Because a long lead time exists between the development of interventions and the resulting improvements in the public's health, an early start on prevention is warranted for most such conditions. Preventive interventions in these areas have been shown to prolong healthy life and reduce expensive hospitalizations. Data suggest that risk factors and disease are more prevalent among the poor than the rich (chapter 7).

- *Con.* In most states, the addition of new programs would divert attention from the unfinished agenda and add complexity to the task of trying to integrate the numerous special programs. Given limited public health capacity and resources, efforts would need to focus on common diseases of childhood and maternity, tuberculosis, and malaria control, which impose a larger burden on the poor. Implementing these programs in the traditional manner, as centrally sponsored schemes, might make it more difficult to undertake other reforms in the national Ministry of Health and Family Welfare and more difficult to organize programs in a state-specific manner.

Action 3: Reduce centrally sponsored schemes and turn over the resources to the states. The central health ministry functions could be refocused on developing policies and plans, allocating funds, and sharing experiences and technical expertise, while management of programs and institutions was devolved to the states and autonomous institutions, as proposed by the Committee on Restructuring the Ministry of Health and Family Welfare (Centre for Policy Research 1999). Centrally sponsored schemes might still be used for experimental activities (for example, the introduction of a public health insurance program), for programs of national interest where public and political awareness is insufficient to ensure adequate attention (for example, HIV control), and for states experiencing special hardships.

- *Pro.* Most centrally sponsored schemes have outlived their purpose. Turning responsibility and resources over to the states would encourage adaptation and innovation in the states, which would be better able to integrate planning and implementation of these schemes with other programs at district and panchayat (a local government administrative body) levels.

- *Con.* Some states might not follow through on implementation of national-priority programs even if the central government retained the ability to monitor progress and influence resource allocation (through the Ministry of Health and Family Welfare and the Planning Commission). Some states might not have the technical capacity to design and implement their own programs, and the central government currently is not organized to provide the type of technical support needed. Resistance to change would be likely within the central bureaucracy, since change would alter roles and reduce central control of resources and influence. Some states also might not want to take up additional responsibilities, as they can now blame insufficient or delayed resources, inappropriate planning and norms, and other inadequacies on the national government (Centre for Policy Research 1999).

Action 4: Reinvest heavily in public health infrastructure and systems. This action would require greater investment in public health and health management training, health information systems, disease surveillance, public health monitoring, and health promotion activities, as proposed in the Bajaj Commission Report (Bajaj 1996).

- *Pro*. Revitalizing public health infrastructure, systems, and human skills would provide a stronger base for public health planning and implementation, areas that are not being filled by the private sector and that have been relatively neglected by the public sector. In the medium to long term, this will be a necessary strategy for providing personnel and systems that are needed to carry out the public health agenda.

- *Con*. With a constrained budget, greater spending on public health might mean lower funding for curative care facilities, a politically sensitive move. Also, some in the public sector would fight measures that empower public health practitioners working in the trenches, wanting instead to preserve planning and information systems that centralize power. For example, shifting the responsibility of the Directorate of Medical Services away from direct administration of hospitals and toward the development of public health policy, the dissemination of health information, and the monitoring public health would likely result in a smaller budget, less purchasing power, and at the least the perception of diminished authority and prestige. More generally, within the medical profession, public health has a lower status than other specialties, and increasing its role might cause friction within existing hierarchies.

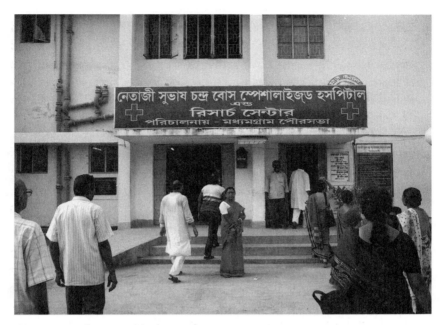

Going to work at a public hospital (PHOTOGRAPH BY GEETANJALI CHOPRA/HEMANT MEHTA/THE WORLD BANK)

Ambulatory Curative Services

Rationale for Public Sector Intervention

Visits for ambulatory curative care account for the great bulk of contacts with the health system, making this an area for public concern. The vast majority of such visits are to the private sector, which includes everything from large, sophisticated hospitals to individuals with no training who dispense dubious or even harmful remedies (chapters 2 and 6).

The rationale for public sector intervention in ambulatory curative services is weaker than in any other area of health care. The case is particularly weak for services that are not related to the treatment of childhood pneumonia or malaria or other such priority programs. Although some externalities exist for nearly any sort of curative care, they are generally not related to public health, and in most instances the benefits are almost entirely private. Since ambulatory curative services have a low cost per episode, the issue of insurance does not loom large. With the increasing burden of chronic disease, however, ambulatory care will become more expensive.

Thus, the public sector arguably needs to play a role in ambulatory curative care because of its supply-side connections with other health activities. For example, curative visits for minor conditions could be used for preventive or promotional activities, and ambulatory curative care visits are part of the chain of referral into more complex care. Credible public preventive services, moreover, may depend on the provision of quality outpatient and inpatient services. However, none of these arguments creates a compelling case for direct public sector production of these health services.

A final argument might be that citizens are entitled to universal availability of a minimal level of curative services. However, such an entitlement is not fulfilled by the current system, nor is it clear why it would be better accomplished through direct production by the public sector versus "demand-side" financing that would allow individuals to choose providers.

Current and Emerging Policy Challenges

The major challenges in service provision are threefold: improving quality, increasing accountability, and promoting equity. Some of the main questions brought out in studies of those challenges are as follows:

- Can government effectively purchase services from the private sector? Can the necessary measurement of performance and costs in the private sector or public sector be created? (chapter 6)

- How can government take advantage of opportunities to work with private providers? Are there opportunities for the public sector to network with alternate private providers by overcoming legal constraints on untrained medical practice? (chapter 6)

- Can government further extend coverage of health services to the poor by encouraging and perhaps formalizing pro-poor measures now being provided by the private sector? Can it effectively monitor health gains by the poor? (chapter 6)

- How can India balance the dual challenges of expanding public spending on critical health services and improving regional equity in resource allocation? (chapter 8)

- How can the experience of stronger states be replicated in poorly performing states to improve health status and reduce polarization? (chapter 9)

Actions for Improving Ambulatory Curative Care

Action 1: Focus public resources strategically in two ways:

   a. Revitalizing public facilities in disadvantaged areas
   b. Purchasing curative care from the private sector when possible.

1a. Revitalizing the network of public sector facilities—but only in disadvantaged areas. Rather than trying to cover the country or all rural areas with rigid input- and population-based norms, government would focus on raising the quality of public sector facilities only where nongovernmental and qualified private sector providers have not been forthcoming.

- *Pro.* This option offers some of the advantages of saving on scarce public sector management capacity while at the same time not withdrawing essential services for which no substitute exists. Under the current approach, in which the government tries to achieve universal coverage following rigid norms, the remote and rural areas already end up with low-quality care, while in urban and densely populated areas the public clinics simply compete, often unsuccessfully, with other providers.

- *Con.* This option has some of the political disadvantages of any attempt to reallocate public sector staff. Stiff political resistance could be expected from health care workers who prefer living in urban areas. The option would be seen as a retreat from a commitment to provide universal basic care.

1b. Purchasing ambulatory curative care from the private sector where possible, and limit its provision from primary health centers (PHCs) and subcenters in those areas. This option would involve moving critical functions such as prenatal care and family planning to public procurement via private sector providers, at least where private sector providers exist and could be demonstrated to be of good quality.

- *Pro.* The main benefit would lie in conserving scarce public sector resources by closing or contracting out underutilized facilities. Because at present only a small fraction of curative care visits are made to government-run facilities, individuals would be able to find other sources of care in nearly all instances of such closures. Most important would be the gain in reorienting the attention and efforts of existing personnel to core public health functions, freeing them from responsibility for curative care while taking advantage of the large private sector in ambulatory care.

- *Con.* The major drawback would be that in some areas—particularly in remote and rural regions—it might be difficult to identify private providers of good quality. Curtailing ambulatory curative care would obviously be a politically unpopular option, one likely to face stiff opposition from public health workers.

Action 2: Expand ambulatory curative care coverage for the poor through the use of "demand-side" mechanisms that give publicly subsidized discounts to the poorest patients at either public or certified private providers. Chapter 6 shows many private sector providers claim to give a variety of discounts to poorer customers. One way to ensure access for the poor is to build on such ad hoc mechanisms by allowing some direct reimbursement to private providers for services provided to poor clients, preferably through mechanisms that allow clients a choice among providers.

- *Pro.* First, reimbursement schemes provide a voluntary linkage between public and private providers. To be eligible for reimbursement, private providers would have their quality of care certified. Second, reimbursement would help redirect poorer households from the lowest-quality providers (untrained private providers) toward higher-quality providers by reducing the costs of the higher-quality private providers. Third, in areas having a large number of certified providers, the public sector could move away from provision altogether, allowing it to focus direct public provision on areas where the poor now have few or no health care options.

- *Con.* The reimbursement option would require the public sector to develop significantly greater administrative capacity to link with the private sector. The public sector would have to be able to assess the quality of private sector providers, create criteria for judging which households were eligible for subsidy and for determining which services were eligible for reimbursement (and at what rate), and avoid corruption (in the form of collusion to over-report services provided).[3] Another major question is how the nationally sponsored programs would interact with private and alternative providers in the various states. In some states, centrally sponsored schemes would be carried out through the system of public clinics, whereas in another the same activities might be contracted out to private sector providers if the state had chosen to eliminate universal coverage of facilities.

Action 3: Invest in raising the quality of the entire network of publicly provided ambulatory services, reorganizing for greater efficiency. This option would mean putting money into public sector ambulatory care, notably care delivered at public health centers and subcenters across the board. Because "more money" is not the solution, revitalization would require organizational and management changes to improve efficiency and public responsiveness.

- *Pro.* The benefit would be better care in the health system. If the quality of public facilities were higher and costs were lower than in the private sector, then presumably people would be attracted to the public alternative. In turn, if the public facilities were attracting more visitors, they could better carry out their preventive and promotional functions.

- *Con*. Revitalizing public health facilities would be enormously expensive. First, since the public sector currently accounts for only 20 percent of visits, enormous increases in facilities or in utilization rates would be required to increase the frequency and proportion of contacts between the poor and the public sector. Second, although money is not the only problem, substantial investments would almost certainly be required to upgrade the quality of care sufficiently to enable public centers to attract new patients. Perhaps even more important, such an effort would attract scarce public sector managerial capacity and human resources away from other parts of the health system: public health, quality assurance, and whatever inpatient role the public sector will play. This strategy would do nothing about the main source of outpatient care provision in the public sector.

Inpatient Curative Services and Health Insurance

Rationale for Public Sector Intervention

Even though inpatient curative care has linkages with oversight, public health services, and ambulatory curative care, it is possible to consider its policy options separately. Treatments having a high cost per episode make the expansion of inpatient care dependent upon some mechanism for pooling risks and thereby redistributing financial costs. In most countries, governments have tried to spread risks and subsidize the poor, though the methods tried have been quite different (box 3.4).

The need to reduce the high levels of risk of financial ruin from serious illness makes inpatient care and health insurance an issue of public concern. Another public sector justification is to ensure that hospitalizations are equitably distributed. The expectation that risk pooling can help to strengthen quality assurance, public accounta-

Box 3.4 International Approaches to Spreading Risks and Subsidizing the Poor

To make health financing fair and efficient, countries have gradually developed a variety of systems to pool risks. By pooling risks, the healthy subsidize those who are sick, and the rich subsidize those who are poor. In the examples shown below, cross-subsidies based on risk (a person's level of illness) and income can occur among members of the same pool or through government subsidies to single or multiple pool arrangements. All systems involve prepayment and a separation of contributions from the use of health services.

COUNTRY	FINANCING SYSTEM	RISK POOLING	SUBSIDIZING OF THE POOR
Colombia	Multiple pools: competing social security organizations, municipal health systems, Ministry of Health	Intrapool via non-risk-related contributions; interpool via a central risk equalization fund. Minimum benefits packages are mandatory for all members of all pools.	Intrapool and interpool: salary-related contributions plus explicit subsidy paid to the insurer for the poor to join social security; supply-side subsidy via no-charge services provided by Ministry of Health and municipal health services
Netherlands	Multiple pools: largely competing private social insurance organizations	Intrapool via non-risk-related contributions; interpool via central risk equalization fund.	Risk equalization fund, excluding the rich
Korea, Republic of	Two main pools: national health insurance (covers up to 30% of a member's health expenditures), Ministry of Health	Intrapool via non-risk-related contribution. A single benefit package for all members.	Salary-related contribution plus supply-side subsidy of Ministry of Health services; national health insurance from government allocations.

Box 3.4 (continued)

COUNTRY	FINANCING SYSTEM	RISK POOLING	SUBSIDIZING OF THE POOR
			Public subsidy for insurance for the poor and farmers.
Zambia	Single formal pool: Ministry of Health/Central Board of Health	Intrapool, implied single benefit package for all in the system.	Intrapool via general taxation. A supply-side subsidy via no-charge services provided by Ministry of Health.
Canada	Single pool in each province (with portability across provinces)	Intrapool, single-benefit package for all citizens.	Intrapool via general taxation.

Source: WHO (2000c).

bility, and purchasing of health services adds to the justification for public involvement in health insurance.

The market for health insurance is especially prone to the problem of "adverse selection": if an insurer offers a policy to all who wish to buy it, then those who elect to buy the insurance will be those who think they have more than the average risk. The resulting loss experience of the insurers will cause them to price the policies "too high" (worse than actuarially fair) for a person of typical risk. For insurers to remain financially viable, they must either force consumers to buy as a "pool" (for example, everyone in a given area, everyone in a given occupation, everyone working for the same firm), screen potential buyers, or price their policies "too high."

Governments often address the insurance problem by providing hospital care at less than full cost. As chapter 9 shows, even with public hospitals, many consumers are forced into debt and poverty by the costs of hospitalization. Moreover, chapter 8 shows that increased cost recovery in public hospitals cannot cover their budget without imposing even greater financial burdens on consumers. But nearly everywhere in the developing world, and in most states of India, the low-cost provision of public hospital care causes the benefits of public expenditures to flow mainly to richer households (chapter 7).

Current and Emerging Policy Challenges

Some of the challenges identified for ambulatory care are also relevant when considering questions of quality, accountability, and equity for inpatient care—and are particularly relevant when considering how India as a whole can learn from its better-performing states and address regional equality in resource allocation. Some specific challenges also face this segment of the health system. A "two-tier" system may emerge in which the poor are effectively left out of quality care in the public sector because of low access and low quality and out of the private sector, as well, because of cost.

Plans for care or insurance that attempt to provide the poor with exactly the same quality and quantity of inpatient care as the rich receive run the risk of cost escalation. The questions raised in studies of such challenges include:

- How can public and private health facilities be made more responsive to the needs of their clients? Can client perceptions of providers' manners and skills be incorporated into training and supervision programs to make health providers more responsive? (chapter 6)

- Can governments intervene in areas that would make the biggest difference in motivating health workers, notably training opportunities? (chapter 6)

- How can the distribution of public expenditures be improved so that a greater fraction reaches the poor? (chapter 7)

- How will India take on the task of migrating from out-of-pocket, fee-for-service financing to risk-pooling mechanisms in a weak regulatory environment? (chapter 8)

- How can India strengthen its financing systems to reduce the large financial risks faced by Indians, particularly the poor, when they become ill? (chapter 9)

Actions for Inpatient Care and Health Insurance

Action 1: Encourage multiple insurance pools. Facilitate the creation of private insurance to pay private providers in a regulatory environment that encourages replication of voluntary employer-based or union-based insurance schemes such as the Self-Employed Women's Association (boxes 3.5 and 8.3). Other community financing and public insurance could also be added to increase coverage. The ultimate objective here would be to reach compulsory purchase of insurance, but with choices for all and public subsidies for the poorest.

- *Pro.* An incremental approach that promises universal coverage might be technically feasible and politically popular. This option would preserve the patient's ability to choose insurer and provider and potentially reduce patient hospital costs markedly and lessen inequity.

- *Con.* For this option to work, information systems, quality assurance procedures, administrative systems, and appropriate marketing strategies would need to be developed, all of which would require investments that the government has not made and capacities that it has not had. The costs would likely be substantial. Explicit decisions about the minimum package of benefits, amounts of public funding, and level of cross-subsidization might expose the Ministry of Health to additional political risks and strain its capacity. From the beginning, increased attention would be needed to get the regulatory framework right lest entrenched interests block subsequent reform. India has had little experience with large-scale non-profit health insurance, and government has little capacity to develop or administer its own public insurance. Partitioning of the risk pools along employment lines would leave government to cover those with the greatest risks and least resources, thus requiring more complicated subsidy schemes among insurance plans.

Box 3.5 Health Insurance for the Informal Sector: The SEWA Experience in Gujarat

The Self-Employed Women's Association (SEWA), a trade union of more than 2 million women in the informal sector, is providing health insurance to its members as part of an integrated insurance scheme. The union developed the plan after SEWA members identified illness—their own and that of family members—as the key stress in their lives and the major cause of indebtedness.

The SEWA health insurance scheme functions in coordination with the Life Insurance Company of India and the new India Assurance Company. Members pay an annual premium and receive coverage for maternity benefits, hospitalization for a wide range of diseases, occupation-related illness, and diseases specific to women.

Several problems emerged in the implementation of the plan (administrative snags, the rejection of valid claims, dishonest claims), but SEWA members are joining the scheme in increasing numbers, setting aside their limited earnings well in advance to pay for the annual premium. SEWA members have no expectation of "free" insurance or subsidies.

The major benefit of the insurance scheme has been to provide security to poor women and their families in times of crisis. In addition, it has enhanced health-seeking behavior and has helped workers to increase their savings and plan for the future.

Box 3.5 (continued)

Insurance and the concept of risk pooling was initially an unknown concept, but SEWA members were quick learners. Women barely familiar with the written word quickly learned some key procedures such as the preservation of bills, certificates, medical cards, and so on.

"Normally, when any of us in the family is sick or hospitalized, it is a dark time for us," said a SEWA member. "This time, when I was hospitalized for cerebral malaria, my family was worried but we did not go into debt forever. I had paid my premium so we recovered most of our costs. Who would have dreamed it was possible?"

Action 2: Move toward "single payer" insurance with compulsory purchase of insurance that would reimburse public and private providers neutrally.

- *Pro.* Universal coverage, the ability to control costs, ease of administration compared to other insurance, and ease of regulation compared to other health insurance—all of these are advantages. The collectivist philosophy behind single-payer insurance and the ability to maintain private provision and patient choice of providers might resonate well in India. This type of financing could strengthen efforts to distinguish good-quality providers from bad and could provide a way to influence clinical practices in the direction of public priorities.

- *Con.* Health systems in India are not ready for compulsory single-payer insurance because public and private providers lack the information systems, quality assurance procedures, and administrative systems to operate such a system. Its initial costs would therefore be very high, depending on the benefit package proposed. The public might lack confidence in its administration and be unwilling to pay additionally for it. The rich might prefer private health insurance to subsidizing the poor, and the healthy might not want to contribute if they did not benefit. Introduction would require political leadership, yet the political risks of failure might be quite high. The problem of controlling costs in a predominantly fee-for-service system has yet to be addressed in India.

Action 3: Rely on the introduction of private, voluntary health insurance. Richer households are using public hospitals less and relying more on private hospitals, a trend that is fueling demand for private health insurance targeted primarily to wealthier households. As richer households abandon the public system, political support for public financing erodes. This could lead to a vicious circle in which low and deteriorating quality in the public sector drives middle- and higher-income households into the private market, which would then further undermine fiscal support of public hospitals. Such a development would effectively exclude the poor from quality care, either by pricing them out of the private market or by deteriorating quality and weakening support for public services.

- *Pro.* The benefit of private, voluntary health insurance is that by essentially ignoring the development of private hospitals the public sector would be able to focus resources on basic public health. This is also the path of least change for the existing bureaucracy and directorate, one that would avoid opposition from that quarter.

- *Con.* Inequalities would grow, and costs would escalate, because the insurance that develops in the private sector for richer clients would be impossibly expensive to generalize. The presence of a private market in one regulatory environment would create entrenched interests that resist reform.

Action 4: Strengthen quality of care especially in public secondary hospitals in rural areas but increase cost recovery, with or without prepayment mechanisms to improve equality. In addition to the financing-based options discussed above, hospital systems and management can also be strengthened in a complementary way.

- *Pro.* The existing rural secondary hospitals are underutilized. Experience shows that improving the quality of these public hospitals increases their efficiency while they continue largely to provide services to the poor (Institute of Health Systems 2000). This approach is popular among state bureaucracies and politicians, so ownership is high and implementation relatively good. Cost recovery at such institutions—when accompanied by improved quality—has provided modest but important amounts of money for facility operations, making them more politically and socially acceptable.

- *Con.* Improving quality in rural secondary hospitals can be expensive and requires continued public financial commitment to operation and maintenance—as well as diligence to ensure that appropriate staff are placed at such facilities. Without such efforts, these approaches could not be sustained. Departments of health have no clear advantage in directly administering hospitals, and in the long run the public agencies might be better off supporting such institutions financially but having them managed by private professional groups under the guidance of a public board. User-fee exemptions for the poor are in place, but it is not known how much of a barrier to care such fees have been to the very poor. Prepayment mechanisms hold a promise of reducing catastrophic costs, but they have not yet been tested.

Action 5: Make public hospitals autonomous and fund their services publicly. This type of institutional reform would separate public sector "provision of insurance" from "provision of curative care." The revenues for these autonomous hospitals could be based strictly on reimbursement for care provided through a public sector financing mechanism—but with no explicit insurance premium, as costs would be paid from general revenue.

- *Pro.* Autonomous organization would offer public hospitals the opportunity to be managed more professionally. More explicit purchasing of services could make hospitals more accountable and improve their performance.

- *Con.* Without changes in the legal environment, the freedom to discharge low-performing workers, more measurable social mandates (such as free care for the poor), and sufficient budgets, making public hospitals autonomous might not achieve the savings, efficiencies, or social mandates expected of them. Because governments would be unlikely to allow public hospitals to be closed, market exposure of these institutions would be limited, and an element of "moral hazard" (insulation from the consequences of poor or irresponsible performance) for these hospitals would likely remain. Professional hospital management has not been well developed in India, so that expected management improvements might not be achieved. Bureaucratic opposition to relinquishing control over hospital administration might make such reforms difficult. Opposition from labor unions and doctors could also be anticipated, particularly if the loss of employment or benefits appeared likely.

Concluding Remarks

This chapter outlined several feasible actions for improving four critical activities of the health sector: oversight of the sector, public health services, ambulatory care, and inpatient services and health insurance. Although we presented the broad advantages and disadvantages of each option, we did not analyze them in terms of their applicability to individual states or health care programs. In chapter 4, we examine how to put some of these options together by assessing which actions are more important for states under different conditions and by examining programs that cut across the main activities discussed in this chapter. To stimulate debate, we propose which of the measures ought to be taken forward in the short and medium terms and outline some of the main policy questions needing further investigation.

Notes

1. S. Nandraj, personal communication, 2001.

2. The unqualified offer treatments that are ineffectual or con-traindicated and, by unmonitored overuse of medicines such as antibiotics, further harm public health by increasing drug resistance (Background Papers 6 and 8).

3. However, all of these are skills that the public sector would need to develop in any case if it were to be involved in regulating providers and insurance.

CHAPTER 4

Putting It Together: Raising the Sights of India's Health System

We now look at ways to pull together the various choices addressed in the preceding chapter. First, we examine the choices facing different states. Second, using maternal health care as an example, we see how different visions for the health system affect health services that cut across the sets of activities discussed in the previous chapter. We then offer some specific policy and operational recommendations for ways to think about what short- and medium-term steps can be taken. We conclude by looking how to take forward the policy and research agenda.

Health system reform should generally improve outcomes in an efficient, equitable, accountable, and sustainable manner. On this basis, we propose in this chapter some broad principles for the types of the reform needed in India's health sector. Government ought to play a leading role in reforming the health sector by raising its sights in four ways:

1. Oversee the needs of the entire population by making the health system more pro-poor, gender sensitive, and client friendly and respond to the high burden of preventable diseases borne by the poor, scheduled tribes and castes, and women.

2. Look forward, by preparing for the challenges already posed by the health transition—a shift in the burden of disease, a rise in

the costs of treatment, and the call to develop a health financing system.

3. Remove blind spots by grappling with the challenges of the development of the private sector so the health system can be considered in its entirety.

4. Focus on improving the quality, efficiency, and accountability of health services, both in the public and private sectors.

Different Choices for Different Parts of India

Overall, in our review a recurrent pattern has emerged in which southern and western states tend to have better health outcomes, higher spending on health, greater use of health services, and more equitable distribution of services than other parts of India, particularly the poor north-central states. A summary of health outcomes for the major Indian states is in table 4.1.

Large differences in health service outputs also exist among the major states (table 4.2). In ranking outputs, we considered higher coverage of prenatal care, higher rates of institutional deliveries, and full immunization as desirable. On the other hand, a higher rate of hospitalization is not necessarily desirable or appropriate.[1] Nearly all states have experienced some success in immunization coverage in at least one district (Rajasthan is the sole state in which no district has at least 70 percent coverage) (table 4.2). To a lesser degree, most states also have at least one district with good prenatal care and institutional delivery coverage. Southern and western states each perform above the Indian average in all three indicators, whereas the performance of poor north-central states tends to be below average for all three areas. Orissa, alone among the poor north-central states, has above-average levels for immunization coverage and prenatal care.

These differences suggest that lower-performing districts and states may be able to learn from their better-performing counter-

Table 4.1 Selected Health Status Outcomes in India and Major Indian States, Selected Years, 1992–99

AREA	LIFE EXPECTANCY AT BIRTH, AVERAGE FOR 1992–96 (YEARS)	NEONATAL MORTALITY, 1998–99 (PER 1,000 LIVE BIRTHS)	INFANT MORTALITY RATE, 1998 (PER 1,000 LIVE BIRTHS)	UNDER-FIVE MORTALITY RATE, 1998–99 (PERCENT)	TOTAL FERTILITY RATE, 1997 (PERCENT)	UNDER-WEIGHT CHILDREN, 1998–99 (PERCENT)
India	61	43	72	95	3.3	47
Andhra Pradesh	62	44	66	86	2.5	38
Assam	56	45	78	90	3.2	36
Bihar	59	47	67	105	4.4	54
Gujarat	61	40	64	85	3.0	45
Haryana	64	35	69	77	3.4	35
Karnataka	63	37	58	70	2.5	44
Kerala	73	14	16	19	1.8	27
Madhya Pradesh	55	55	98	138	4.0	55
Maharashtra	65	32	49	58	2.7	50
Orissa	57	49	98	104	3.0	54
Punjab	67	34	54	72	2.7	29
Rajasthan	60	50	83	115	4.3	51
Tamil Nadu	64	35	53	63	2.0	37
Uttar Pradesh	57	54	85	123	4.8	52
West Bengal	62	32	53	68	2.6	49

Note: Major Indian states are those with a population of at least 15 million. Bihar includes Jharkhand, Madhya Pradesh includes Chatisgarh, and Uttar Pradesh includes Uttaranchal. Neonatal mortality is of those less than one month of age; infant mortality is of those less than one year of age; under-five mortality is of those less than five years of age; total fertility rate is lifetime births per woman aged 15–49; underweight children are those under three years of age whose weight is statistically low for their age (that is, more than 2 standard deviations below average).
Source: Registrar General (1999); IIPS (2000).

parts. Differences among states in the degree of equality in the distribution of health services (chapter 7) should also provide good learning opportunities.

Two factors have a major influence on the health systems choices facing each state: (a) the state's position in the health transition and (b) capacity of the state's public health sector. The position of the major states on these two scales is measured according to infant mortality, child mortality, total fertility, and immunization coverage (table 4.3).[2]

Table 4.2 Selected Health Service Outcomes in Major Indian States and India Overall, Selected Years, 1995–99

STATE	FULL PRENATAL CARE, 1999 (PERCENT OF BIRTHS)			INSTITUTIONAL DELIVERIES, 1999 (PERCENT OF BIRTHS)			FULL IMMUNIZATION, 1998–99 (PERCENT OF CHILDREN 1 TO 3 YEARS OLD)			PUBLIC HOSPITALIZATIONS (PER 100,000 PERSONS PER YEAR) 1995–96	PRIVATE HOSPITALIZATIONS (PER 100,000 PERSONS PER YEAR) 1995–96
	STATE AVERAGE	LOWEST DISTRICT	HIGHEST DISTRICT	STATE AVERAGE	LOWEST DISTRICT	HIGHEST DISTRICT	STATE AVERAGE	LOWEST DISTRICT	HIGHEST DISTRICT		
Andhra Pradesh	62	41	82	51	28	88	75	51	91	442	1,153
Assam	24	4	82	24	6	76	47	4	95	200	522
Bihar	10	3	43	15	5	44	22	7	71	539	1,172
Gujarat	36	16	65	46	13	68	58	21	76	905	1,946
Haryana	21	15	37	26	17	43	66	47	90	2,206	270
Karnataka	59	27	88	50	18	83	72	25	95	2,944	4,536
Kerala	85	68	92	97	88	100	84	60	97	581	448
Madhya Pradesh	17	2	53	22	7	62	48	11	90	792	1,727
Maharashtra	49	30	81	57	16	93	80	59	94	1,168	223
Orissa	32	17	61	23	7	57	58	28	80	1,162	158
Punjab	18	14	41	41	25	58	73	52	94	530	1,092
Rajasthan	15	5	30	23	7	37	37	12	60	669	336
Tamil Nadu	75	46	95	79	55	99	92	77	100	848	1,290
Uttar Pradesh	11	4	67	16	5	43	44	3	82	440	565
West Bengal	33	16	53	39	20	91	52	29	83	1,088	353
All states in India	28	2	95	34	5	100	54	3	100	726	928

Note: Major states are those with a population of more than 15 million. Bihar includes Jharkhand, Madhya Pradesh includes Chatisgarh, and Uttar Pradesh includes Uttaranchal.

Source: IIPS (1998–99); National Sample Survey Organisation (1998).

The ability of governments to oversee the health sector or to inform and influence the public has not been the dominant feature of government actions in the public sector, so it is not explicitly measured for the ranking of state capacity. The capacity and scope of the private sector also influences the range of options available to the state. At this point, however, we can distinguish only between the levels of involvement of the private sector in the states and not between the differences in quality of services or cohesiveness of organization.[3] As chapter 7 notes, high levels of private sector hospitalization are associated with a more pro-poor distribution of public hospitalization, a fact suggesting that states are better able to concentrate public resources on delivering services to the poor when the private sector is more active.[4]

States differ in their position within the health transition. A state such as Kerala already faces the burden of how to deal with high-cost-per-episode health care. Whatever capacity Kerala has developed to deliver public services, it must now meet the new chal-

Table 4.3 Categorization of Major Indian States by Characteristics Influencing Fundamental Health System Choices

CHARACTERISTIC OF STATE	STATES	PERCENT OF INDIA'S POPULATION (2001)
A. Middle to late transition, moderate to high capacity	Kerala, Tamil Nadu	9.1
B. Early to middle transition, low to moderate capacity	Maharashtra, Karnataka, Punjab, West Bengal, Andhra Pradesh, Gujarat, Haryana	39.1
C. Very early to early transition, very low to low capacity	Orissa, Rajasthan, Madhya Pradesh, Uttar Pradesh	33.1
D. Special cases of instability: high to very high mortality plus civil conflict or very poor governance, or both	Assam, Bihar	13.3

Note: Major states (those having a population of more than 15 million) were ranked according to rates of infant mortality, child mortality, total fertility, and full immunization. The estimates were made before bifurcation, so Bihar includes Jharkhand, and Madhya Pradesh includes Chattisgarh, and Uttar Pradesh includes Uttaranchal.

lenges without having developed the type of systems needed to face them—systems such as risk-pooling financing systems, information systems on provider performance, and mechanisms to take full advantage of networks of private and public providers. Indeed, as shown in part II, these systems are lacking throughout India. Kerala's public health and preventive programs also need to respond to a shifting burden of disease and rising public demands.

States like Orissa or Madhya Pradesh, on the other hand, are at the other end of India's health transition. They must focus on pre-transition diseases by implementing the public programs needed to prevent and diminish these conditions. In such states, building the government's capacity to measure outpatient and hospital perform-ance and to develop health financing systems are important, but they are less important right now than improving the quality and reach of the current priority public programs. Although states in the pre-transition phase (categories C and D in terms of table 4.3), like those further along, need partnerships between the public and private sec-tors, the focus of such efforts must be less on hospitalization and financing systems and more on basic public health services.[5] States in category B, by contrast, must adjust to the health transition by shifting their emphasis on systems, capacities, and content of pro-grams; their challenge is to decide when and how to start doing so.

Many other factors also influence the choices to be made between and within states, some of which are outlined in table 4.4. The large urban municipalities need to simplify the overlap and confusion of public providers, systematically work with the dominant private sec-tors, reduce the harmful effects of pollution, and develop more extensive services for the urban poor. Some of these steps have been taken in projects such as the Calcutta Urban Slums Project, but none has focused on making urban services more comprehensive and coherent.

Geographic factors distinguish conditions in mountainous states such as Uttaranchal and Himachal Pradesh. These states have been quite diligent and creative in providing outreach health services, but their problems with transport and access to primary curative and first

Table 4.4 Local Factors to Consider at State Level when Prioritizing Health Systems Choices

LOCAL FACTOR	EXAMPLES
Lifestyle differences	• Nonsmoking tobacco use is 25 times greater in Orissa than in Haryana • Smoking rates are 3.4 times greater in West Bengal than in Maharashtra • Alcohol use is 5 times greater in Madhya Pradesh than in Haryana
Poverty differentials	• Large differences between northeast Karnataka and south Karnataka; and in Maharashtra State between Mumbai and rural areas
Natural risks	• Flooding in Ganges delta, drought in Rajasthan • Cyclones in Orissa, Andhra Pradesh, and West Bengal • Earthquakes in Gujarat and Uttaranchal
Physical environment	• Slums and pollution around megacities • Indoor air pollution (fuel combustion) in rural households • Mountain isolation in Uttaranchal and Himachal Pradesh
Political outlook	• Communist and collectivist philosophies in Kerala and West Bengal • Greater decentralization and stronger local bodies in Kerala and Madhya Pradesh
Social capital	• Large numbers of NGOs and community groups in Gujarat

referral care are more daunting than elsewhere and justify a higher priority for public infrastructure in such remote areas. The island territories also have special needs. Some states are especially vulnerable to natural risks such as flooding and cyclones, making preparedness for such disasters a more important factor than elsewhere in shaping health systems.

Large differences in health risks arising from lifestyle patterns should also be considered. According to the 1995–96 National Sample Survey (NSSO 1998), which surveyed people aged 10 years or older, regular use of nonsmoking tobacco ranges from less than 3 percent in Haryana and Uttar Pradesh to more than 40 percent in Orissa.[6] On the other hand, the prevalence of tobacco smoking is less than 8 percent in Maharashtra and Punjab and goes as high as 27 percent among the northeast states and 24 percent in West Bengal. The prevalence of regular alcohol consumption is as high as 11.5

percent in the northeast and 8.6 percent in Madhya Pradesh, compared with less than 2 percent in Uttar Pradesh and Haryana.

Men and women also differ in their lifestyle risks (men have much higher rates of use of tobacco and alcohol), as do people at different income levels (see chapter 7). For those below the poverty line in India, the prevalence of regular use of nonsmoking tobacco is 37 percent higher than for those above the poverty line, 8 percent higher for smoking, and 28 percent higher for alcohol consumption. The poor are therefore more likely than those with higher incomes to suffer the negative health consequences of these behaviors. In states where the risks are higher, considerations of efficiency as well as equity suggest that preparation for dealing with these high-cost illnesses should come sooner rather than later.

Choices for the Central Government

The central government has important options for deploying its resources and for arranging its relationships with the states in addressing programs of national importance such as health care. Yet a high-powered advisory committee from the Centre for Policy Research (CPR), entrusted to consider "Restructuring the Ministry of Health and Family Welfare," noted that no previous attempt had been made to define the appropriate role for the Health Ministry in the Indian federal system (Centre for Policy Research 1999). The CPR report held that the central government has taken a role in health care that has gone beyond that envisioned in the Constitution. In doing so, the central government has assumed overly centralized control of health and family welfare programs and of executive and regulatory functions, created overly rigid planning procedures and standards for its programs, and weakened policymaking and innovation at the state level.

Rather than provide options, the CPR report emphatically recommended that the core functions of the central ministry be defined around a set of national responsibilities for policy, planning, and monitoring, while the responsibilities for the allocation of resources

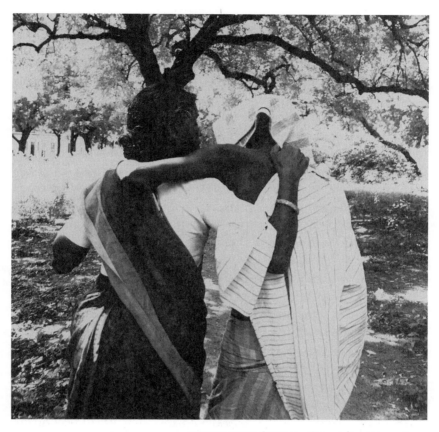

PHOTOGRAPH BY GEETANJALI CHOPRA/THE WORLD BANK

and executive functions are delegated to state governments and fully autonomous organizations. For the ministry to fulfill the proposed core functions, the report recommended a specific and challenging list of reforms, many of which would strengthen the central government's oversight capacity while hastening the prescribed devolution to the states.[7] If the central government were to take on this ambitious agenda, it would have little time for other activities in the short term. In the long run, however, the payoff could be quite large: the ministry would be more cohesive and efficient, and many of the new functions proposed are currently neglected but vital to the role the central government will need to play in the future.

The importance of centrally sponsored schemes to the health profile of India (see chapter 7) and the problems with the current implementation arrangements in many of the programs mean that decentralization of these programs will be difficult, even if not taken to the extent advocated in the CPR report. Some steps have already been taken in the Leprosy Elimination Program, which features state plans that vary on the basis of the local prevalence of the disease and the ability of the state to provide supporting systems such as information technology, planning and budgeting, and logistics. Programs also exist for reproductive and child health and for the control of AIDS, tuberculosis, and malaria. As in the case of the leprosy program, these efforts must consider the variations in health status in the states and the feasibility of integrating the programs with supporting systems and general health services.

The central government's role in setting service norms also deserves reconsideration. For decades, centrally mandated national norms for public health infrastructure have dominated policy discussion and public effort (Duggal 2000; Centre for Policy Research 1999). Yet rigid input norms have been unrelated to workload, local epidemiological conditions, and the presence of a private sector that is the main provider of outpatient and inpatient care. The norms thus create large distortions and inefficiencies, and the centralized approach is less relevant today than ever before.

Seven states have attempted to rationalize their public service norms (for services, staff, drugs, and equipment) to better match their capacity to deliver with the presence of the private sector, and different needs across the state.[8] These efforts have largely focused on much neglected secondary services and have been part of broader investments to improve referral systems and the quality of services. This type of exercise needs to be continually updated as experience is gained to ensure that high-quality services are being sustained and that the public and providers are satisfied with the scope and performance of health services. The approach is also worthwhile extending across all levels of care and in other states and could provide a basis for using standards in the private sector as well. The central government could facilitate this process by bringing together the lessons learned across the country.

Guidance from the central government may now be more important than ever as the need for new areas of government intervention becomes clear. For example, guidance on quality standards and processes in health care is relevant for both the public and private sectors, but it is sorely lacking. Sharing of information and analyses of health system financing, outputs, and outcomes across states and districts is also needed if lessons are to be learned and successful practices emulated. Existing areas of involvement in oversight functions also need to be strengthened. Examples include the use of the Medical Certificate of Cause of Death and the Survey of Cause of Death. Expanded investment in health information systems by the central government should be considered even if it means reducing the curative services the central government finances.

Whether the central government takes on these oversight tasks itself or finances others to do them, it will have to acquire for itself new skills, systems, and behaviors. Refocusing its efforts presumably implies a reduction in the other activities that currently take up its energies, such as the operation of national institutions, advancement of the Central Government Health Scheme, the management of centrally sponsored schemes, and the recurrent high profile health emergencies that are raised in Parliament or the media.

Chapter 8 points out that many options also exist for determining the future of central financing of health. Although central spending on health is currently relatively minor (about 23 percent of public spending on health), it provides important funds for priority programs, in some cases replacing what states might otherwise spend on them. However, questions remain as to whether central funds should be given equally to states (for example, on a per capita basis); used to equalize public spending among states; used to provide extra funds for states with special needs (for example, states with poor health conditions, poor health infrastructure, or those having a disaster); or provided to those states that perform better or take up important innovations (for example, states that implement a centrally sponsored scheme particularly well or introduce a new scheme, such as hepatitis B vaccine or public health insurance).

The central government also has choices to make about how it wishes to intervene in particular states, especially those identified as having special needs (category D in table 4.3). The options for intervention in such states represent a special case for the central government in part because of the high level of health needs in those states; the size of their population; and the breakdown in governance, including the public health sector. The Action Plan for the National Population Policy (Ministry of Health and Family Welfare 2000b) established an Empowered Action Group to provide the necessary resources and organizational force to improve health conditions in Bihar and four other poorly performing states (Madhya Pradesh, Orissa, Rajasthan, and Uttar Pradesh). Although building local capabilities through the central government is necessary in the long run, other options for the financing and management of programs should be considered for the short to medium term in states such as Bihar and others having special needs. One option is to have a greater role for direct central government financing and management of health and family welfare programs. This option may be realized by pay to have the management and delivery of services handled by a third party such as a new society, a nonprofit NGO, a private company, or an international agency.[9]

Choices for the States

The differences among states should mean that states have different priorities. In table 4.3, position in the health transition and the state government's capabilities were proposed as major points of differentiation among states, along with other features specific to the various states (in table 4.4).

Recalling the options for the four critical areas of health care activity discussed in chapter 3, we now propose a set of options that are facing the states in different categories as well as the central government (table 4.5). Since international experience suggests that the need to evaluate

Table 4.5 Major Health System Choices Facing Indian States, by Stage of the Health Transition, and the Central Government

STATE CATEGORY	HEALTH SYSTEM OVERSIGHT	PUBLIC HEALTH SERVICES	AMBULATORY CURATIVE CARE	INPATIENT CARE	HEALTH FINANCING
A. Middle to late transition, moderate to high capacity	• How to instill quality assurance for public and private sectors • How to measure and disseminate performance of private and public sectors • Types of partnership with private sector that can be implemented (contracting, cooperation, etc.)	• How to introduce and expand programs for heart disease, injuries, mental health, and HIV	• How to build networks with private providers • How to "contract" with private sector • Whether to reduce direct public provision, more selectivity in services provided (e.g. prenatal care) or focus on backward areas	• Whether and how to move from public provision to public insurance • How to "contract" with private sector • Whether and how to strengthen publicly run hospitals serving rural areas	• How to introduce health insurance with universal coverage • How to raise more resources for health. • How to test demand-side financing for priority curative care (ambulatory and inpatient)
B. Early to middle transition, low to moderate capacity	• How to inform and empower people to demand better health services • Types of partnership with private sector can be implemented (contracting, cooperation, etc.)	• When and how to introduce programs for heart disease, injuries, mental health, and HIV	• How to build networks with private providers • Whether to refocus public outpatient care only in backward areas or across state	• Whether and how to move from public provision to public insurance • How to "contract" with private sector • Whether and how to strengthen publicly run hos-	• When and how to introduce health insurance by experimentation • How to test demand-side financing for priority curative care

(Table continues on the following page.)

Table 4.5 (continued)

STATE CATEGORY	HEALTH SYSTEM OVERSIGHT	PUBLIC HEALTH SERVICES	AMBULATORY CURATIVE CARE	INPATIENT CARE	HEALTH FINANCING
C. Very early to early transition, very low to low capacity	• How to inform and empower people to demand better health services • How to bring public and private sector actors together to work on common interests	• How to better inform and empower people to live more healthfully, focusing on pre-transition conditions and HIV	• Whether and how to work with untrained practitioners • How to rejuvenate public facilities in backward areas or across state	pitals serving rural areas • How to put appropriate balance on primary, secondary, and tertiary care	• Whether to test small demand-side financing for priority curative care, especially where the private sector is large
D. National government	• How to refocus on national oversight issues, promoting quality assurance in public and private sectors; national-level information, education, and communications; information on health system performance; drug quality control	• How to devolve centrally sponsored schemes to states and local bodies to facilitate better implementation • How to intervene in very poorly performing states (e.g. Bihar) or states in special circumstances (Jammu and Kashmir)	• Whether and how to develop standards and accreditation and licensing schemes • Whether and how to develop guidelines, training, and patient education materials	• Whether and how to provide examples for how to reorganize large hospitals • Whether and how to provide incentives for development of provider networks	• Whether to raise more funds for health (e.g. through general revenues or tobacco or alcohol taxes) • Whether to use central funds to counteract inter-state differences in public financing, health needs, or performance • Whether and how to stimulate public health insurance

the health system and improve it is continuous, the suggestions outlined in table 4.5 should be considered a work in progress. The purpose of presentation here is not so much to limit the options for specific states but to provide additional substance to the debate and suggest which set of options may be tackled first by states having different conditions.

Health System Oversight

In the long run, all states ought to be able to deliver on each of the actions in table 4.6 for improving oversight. Each state ought to develop its health policy to be more comprehensive in its scope and initiate steps to improve measurability in the private sector. The difference between what states can do and should do may be more dependent on opportunities that are available, leadership that emerges in the states, and the urgency of the issues.

States in categories A and B in table 4.3 (especially mid-late transition, moderate-high capacity) need to institutionalize quality assurance procedures in inpatient and ambulatory services through a balanced approach of options involving providers and consumers (actions 1 through 6). Perhaps the best way to start is with action 2, using independent organizations to measure performance because the problems of credibility and conflict may be larger at the beginning of these reforms. However, action 2 may require the development of considerable trust between public and private sectors, which could be accomplished through the promotion of partnerships between the public and private sectors (action 1). Increasing the role of consumer advocates is another good approach to strengthening oversight (action 4).

For other states, focusing initial activities on empowering people to demand better health services and initiating steps to bring together actors from the public and private sectors may be more feasible (actions 1 and 3). As experience and confidence is gained, more actions could be pursued.

Public Health Services

Clear differences exist between the states in the area of public health services. States in category A have a more compelling reason to focus

Table 4.6 Pros and Cons of Actions for Improving Oversight

ACTION	PROS	CONS
1. Develop partnerships with the private sector to share information, improve quality, cooperate on service provision.	• Potential for improving information, efficiency, and coverage of services. • Contracting has potential for increased accountability and efficiency.	• Difficult with low measurability of services and unclear social mandates. • Requires capacity in public sector to manage contracts. • Potential for increased conflict among competing providers. • Shortage of qualified providers in rural areas may persist.
2. Support independent organizations to measure performance among public and private providers.	• Credibility of honest broker. • Potentially efficient way to address information and quality assurance needs.	• Difficult to maintain independence. • Needs goodwill from public and private sector. • Potentially threatening to public and private sectors.
3. Support professional self-regulation.	• Likely to gain support from private sector.	• Little credibility to consumers or government as an honest broker. • Technical capacity has not been tested.
4. Facilitate consumer health advocacy organizations independent of both public providers and private associations.	• Potential to increase people's participation. • Low-cost way to raise accountability and performance of the health system.	• Few organizations have capacity. • Requires investment in their development. • Risk of advocacy groups being "captured" by political and other interest groups. • Consumer groups typically represent middle and upper classes; may not take on interests of the poor.
5. Establish or strengthen formal regulation of health inputs such as pharmaceuticals.	• Addresses major problems with drug quality control. • Current system underfinanced.	• Little capacity in public sector to effectively regulate. • Risks creating inspectorate raj.

6. Establish formal public sector regulation of private providers through legislation.	• Addresses problems of untrained practitioners and harmful medical practices. • Gives teeth to current weak system.	• Same as in action 5 above, but more difficult to measure objectively • Risk of "regulatory capture," limited competition, and higher prices. • Creates adversarial relationship between regulators and providers.

Table 4.7 Pros and Cons of Actions for Improving Public Health Services

ACTION	PROS	CONS
1. Concentrate effort on programs for the "unfinished agenda" by increasing funding and increasing effectiveness	• Addresses major burden of disease • Highly cost-effective interventions exist. • Programs already exist.	• Existing programs are overly centralized and have weak management capacity, and do not have the political support to make them work as well as they should. • The reforms needed in these programs may not be forthcoming. • Costs of these programs may require tradeoffs which may reduce funds for curative care and raise political risks and opposition from staff.
2. Initiate and strengthen programs in noncommunicable diseases in states well advanced in the epidemiological transition	• Will address a burden of disease that is large and growing • Will help develop programs that are small and underfunded • Effective preventive interventions will prolong healthy lives and reduce expensive hospitalizations in the future. • For states well into the health transition, the poor will benefit disproportionately from such measures.	• May distract attention from the "unfinished agenda," especially in states that are in early stages of the health transition and have little capacity to develop and implement new programs • May be implemented as traditional centrally sponsored scheme, making it more difficult to undertake other reforms in the national MOHFW or organize programs in a state-specific manner
3. Reduce centrally sponsored schemes, turn over the resources to the states, and reassign functions of national MOHFW	• Reduces problems with national norms and dependence on center • Increases the role of states, so that planning and accountabilities are closer to the level of implementation • Should encourage adaptation to local needs and innovation by states	• Some states may not follow through on implementation of national priority programs. • Some states do not have technical capacity to design and implement their own programs. • Some states may not want additional responsibilities, since they can now blame national government for inadequacies.

	• Should encourage greater integration of public programs • Allows national MOHFW to focus on policy, information sharing, technical guidance, and issues of national importance, which currently receive insufficient attention	• National MOHFW is not organized to provide the technical support needed by states. • Risk of resistance by national bureaucracy and politicians, since change entails loss of control of resources and direct influence and reduces opportunities for promotion • Untested mechanisms for national MOHFW to appropriately monitor progress and influence resource allocation under new arrangements
4. Reinvest heavily in public health systems—institutions, management information systems, surveillance	• Leads to stronger skills base • More effective health planning, implementation, and monitoring • Private sector is not addressing this area, and it has been neglected by public sector.	• Costs may involve tradeoffs which may reduce funds for curative care and raise political risks and opposition from staff. • Little current capacity in training institutions • Risks opposition in directorates of health, as powers shift to public health, with increased information flow and less direct control over hospital budgets and purchase of supplies • Potential opposition from non–public-health medical specialties

Note: MOHFW, Ministry of Health and Family Welfare.

on introducing and expanding public health services for cardiovascular disease, mental health, and injuries, as these are now the prominent conditions facing their populations (action 2 in table 4.7). States in category B may be in the position of considering when and how to introduce these programs, as these threats loom large in the near future. States in table 4.3 in category C, such as Orissa, in which tobacco chewing is widespread, may need to consider putting more effort into public health campaigns related to lifestyle-related health problems; but in the main, states in categories C and D will want to focus on improving implementation of the existing public health programs that tackle the conditions of the "unfinished agenda," notably reproductive and child health, nutrition, and tuberculosis control (action 1) along with investments in sanitation and water. These options could be implemented through action 3 (provide resources to the state and convert the role of the central government's Ministry of Health and Family Welfare).

All states need to put additional resources into HIV prevention, although the mix of interventions may vary from state to state. Each state and the central government may find that action 4 (reinvest in general public health systems) is also an important means of implementing any public health strategy in the medium to long term. In any event, the success of public health programs usually depends on more than funding the technical interventions, as demonstrated in an analysis of recent "success stories" in low-income countries (box 4.1).

Ambulatory Care

Using the options for ambulatory curative care discussed in chapter 3 (shown in this chapter in table 4.8), the higher-capacity states (categories A and B) may wish to move toward something like a combination of action 1 (revitalizing public facilities in disadvantaged areas and purchasing services from private providers) and action 2 (demand-side mechanisms for the poor); such an approach suggests itself because the health sector in the category A and B states is sufficiently developed so that the presence or absence of a public facility would make a difference only in remote areas, and these states would have the ability to form linkages with the private sector to protect the poor.

Box 4.1 Keys to Success

Many low-income countries have shown that if they use the available tools both widely and wisely, health outcomes can be improved dramatically. Many countries have success stories in spite of poverty. Malawi is set to eliminate measles despite the fact that only 3 percent of the population has access to adequate sanitation, and Bangladesh has reduced neonatal tetanus fatalities by more than 90 percent even though most mothers in the country do not have access to a clean delivery environment. The keys to these successes seem to be political commitment, the development of public-private partnerships, a willingness to innovate, health education, and measurability in programs. Several of these factors seem to have been at work in the successes being realized by Malawi and Bangladesh; additional country examples are given in the following elaboration of these keys to success.

Political Commitment

Efforts to reduce the burden of disease have been driven by a firm political commitment. Examples include Uganda and Thailand, where political leadership has been critical in the fight against HIV/AIDS. Another example is Peru, where the government has established the control of tuberculosis as a social, political, and economic priority.

Partnerships

Success has involved partnerships with the private sector and NGOs for the social marketing of condoms in Uganda and for malaria control in Azerbaijan. In some countries, governments are providing health services and commodities outside the formal sector in an effort to broaden access to health care. In Senegal, mosques throughout the country

Box 4.1 (continued)

are a focal point for HIV prevention efforts, counseling, and support. In Tanzania, a school-based program has improved the health of children with intestinal worms, and in Kenya, employers are supplying bednets to their work force through payroll purchasing schemes.

Innovation

Innovation, born of a pragmatic approach to achieving results, has made a difference. In Nepal, accommodations in hostels are provided to TB patients from remote mountain areas to encourage their compliance with treatment. In Thailand, the government worked with brothel owners to spread the use of condoms—despite the fact that prostitution remains illegal.

Health Education

Health education and training of extension health care workers have been key elements for success. In Sri Lanka, high female literacy rates and midwifery training for health care workers have both been instrumental in preventing maternal deaths. Sex education for children and adolescents has been an integral part of successful HIV prevention programs in Thailand, Senegal, and Uganda.

Measurability

Measuring outcomes is central to the development of successful programs. In Senegal, Thailand, and Uganda, systems of disease surveillance and monitoring have been essential to tracking the course of the HIV/AIDS epidemic and to monitoring the effectiveness of interventions.

Source: WHO (2000a).

Table 4.8 Pros and Cons of Actions for Improving Ambulatory Curative Care

ACTION	PROS	CONS
1. Focus public resources strategically by (a) Revitalizing the network of public sector facilities—but only in disadvantaged areas where private sector and NGO alternatives are not available. (b) Limiting the provision of ambulatory curative care by PHCs and subcenters wherever such care is available from the private sector.	• Realizes some savings in scarce public funds and management capacity. • Improves quality of public services where they are most important. • Focuses public resources on areas of need and reduces inflexible application of norms. • Saves resources by closing underutilized facilities. • Potentially reorients staff back to core public health services. • Takes advantage of large private sector.	• Some political opposition if seen as a retreat from universal care. • Potential for nontransparent manipulation for selection of disadvantaged areas. • Opposition from public sector staff who may need to be moved from urban areas and hospitals to rural primary care facilities. • Politically unpopular if seen as a retreat from public commitment to health. • Public sector workers likely to oppose change in roles and potential loss of jobs. • Some rural areas may have no quality private providers available. • Difficult to identify private providers of good quality.
2. Expand ambulatory curative care coverage for the poor through demand-side mechanisms that give the poorest patients access to publicly subsidized discounts from public or certified private providers.	• Builds on a voluntary linkage between public and private providers. • Provides an entrée for meaningful quality assurance, if providers need to have "certified" quality of care to be eligible for reimbursement. • Helps redirect poorer households from untrained practitioners to higher-quality providers. • Allows public sector to more easily move out of provision in areas where there are good private alternatives.	• Requires greater commitment of public sector to build administrative capacity to link with the private sector. • Capacity needed to assess quality of private providers, create criteria for household eligibility, define service packages and reimbursement rates, and avoid corruption (collusion and overreporting of services). This has not been tested. • Priority centrally sponsored schemes requiring clinical services may have very different approaches with public and private clinics across states, testing the flexibility of the central government • In some rural areas no quality private providers may be available.

(Table continues on the following page.)

Table 4.8 (continued)

ACTION	PROS	CONS
	• Allows public sector provision to be concentrated in areas where poor have fewer options. • Because many private providers already provide discounts to the poor, option would build on current experience.	• High costs; needed funds have not come in the past. • The needed organizational reforms have always been limited. • Scarce public sector managerial capacity would be diverted from other parts of the health system: public health services, oversight, quality assurance, inpatient care, and development of new financing systems.
3. Invest in raising quality of the entire network of publicly provided ambulatory services, reorganizing for greater efficiency.	• Potential for increased quality of care. • Could attract more poor people currently using low-quality private care to use public facilities. • More opportunities to carry out preventive and promotional services. • Maintains current balance of interests, preventing opposition from those who may not gain if more selective improvements are made.	• The private sector would still provide the bulk of services nationwide and to the poor; the effect of these actions upon the poor is probably limited.

Note: PHCs, primary health centers.

In the low- and very-low-capacity states (categories C and D) that still have high rates of infant mortality and low coverage of basic public health measures such as immunizations and nutrition programs, a different approach would make sense. These states would de-emphasize publicly provided ambulatory curative care, emphasizing instead action 1a (reducing public ambulatory curative care at non-hospital facilities) and action 1b (concentrating public facilities in disadvantaged areas) to allow a reallocation of effort to public health activities. These actions may be more viable in states with greater private provision of outpatient services, although the fear of political repercussions may prevent such approaches, especially for action 1b. If a windfall of resources were to become available, action 4 (revitalize the entire network of public facilities) would become more attractive.

The states with medium capacity and medium health performance (category B) face the largest strategic issue: because the private sector may still be underdeveloped and the treatable conditions of the "unfinished agenda" may constitute a large component of mortality, they might want to invest in the creation of a well functioning public ambulatory curative care system (action 3). On the other hand, since the private sector delivers most ambulatory curative care, they may want to skip that effort entirely and move to the creation of more links with the private sector (action 2).

Inpatient Care and Health Insurance

The states in categories A and B must pay considerable attention to inpatient care and health insurance because high-cost care consumes a large part of the health expenditures in these states. Forward-looking states in categories A and B should be concerned about choosing between action 1 (multiple public and private health insurers) and action 2 (universal public insurance) as outlined in table 4.9. Nonetheless, no state is in a position to introduce major health insurance without first doing the careful groundwork that is needed to make these efforts successful. The groundwork includes public consensus-building and policy decisions; addressing the level of prepayment for insurance, the mechanisms for pooling funds, and the man-

Table 4.9 Pros and Cons of Actions for Improving Inpatient Care and Health Insurance

ACTION	PROS	CONS
1. Encourage multiple insurance pools. Facilitate the creation of private insurance to pay private providers in a regulatory environment that encourages replication of voluntary employer or union-based insurance schemes (such as the Self-Employed Women's Association) along with public insurance	• An incremental approach that holds out the promise of universal care may be technically feasible and politically popular. • Preserves choice of provider and insurer and has the potential to reduce catastrophic costs and inequality if done well	• The necessary information systems, quality assurance procedures, administrative systems, and marketing strategies are undeveloped. • Will require investments that the government has not made in the past, and the costs are likely to be substantial • Explicit decisions about the minimum package of benefits, amounts of public funding, and level of cross-subsidization may expose the national MOHFW to additional political risks and overtax its capacity. • The regulatory framework is not yet in place, so that interests may become entrenched and block subsequent reforms. • India has little experience with nonprofit health insurance of sufficient scale, and government has little capacity to develop or administer its own public insurance. • Partitioning of the risk pools along lines of employment leaves government to cover those with the greatest risks and least resources, requiring more complicated subsidy schemes among insurance plans. • Most of the population work in the informal sector and is difficult to include in these schemes.
2. Move toward compulsory purchase of "single payer" insurance that reimburses public and private providers neutrally	• Universal coverage, ability to control costs, ease of administration compared to other insurance options. • Collectivist approach and ability to	• Public and private providers do not have the necessary information systems, quality assurance procedures, and administrative systems. • The costs are likely to be initially very high, depending

110

Strategy	Advantages	Disadvantages
(continued from previous page)	maintain private provision and patient choice may give this popular appeal. • Can be used to improve quality assurance and influence clinical practices in line with public priorities	on the benefit package proposed. • The public may lack confidence in administration of scheme and be unwilling to increase payment for public insurance. • The rich may prefer private health insurance to subsidizing the poor, and the healthy may not want to contribute if they do not benefit. • Requires political leadership, yet the political risks of failure may be quite high. • The problem of controlling costs in a predominantly fee-for-service system has not yet been addressed.
3. Rely on the introduction of private voluntary health insurance	• Public sector may be able to focus resources on public health by spending less attention on hospitals. • Path of least resistance in health care financing reform	• Escalation of the cost of health services to consumers • Increased inequalities: If richer households use the public system less, there will be even less political support for public financing of public hospitals and a vicious circle of declining quality and fewer middle- and upper-income patients. • The private market is difficult to regulate; creates entrenched interests that resist reform.
4. Strengthen quality of care, especially in public sector secondary hospitals serving rural areas, but increase cost recovery with or without prepayment mechanisms to improve equality	• Would take advantage of under-utilized public hospitals • Positive experience in state health systems' development projects • Approach is popular with state politicians and bureaucracy, so commitment is relatively high. • Cost recovery at these institutions has been associated with quality	• Requires considerable resources and continued financial commitment for operation and maintenance, none of which was available in the past • Staff and politicians resist reforms in staff placement. • State departments of health may not have the capacity to directly administer hospitals. • User-fee exemptions for the poor are in place, but it is not known how much of a barrier to care such fees have been.

(Table continues on the following page.)

Table 4.9 (continued)

ACTION	PROS	CONS
	improvements and provided important flexible funds for operations, making fees socially and politically feasible.	• Approach is insufficient to address issues of reducing catastrophic costs to patients, as no prepayment and risk pooling have been attempted.
5. Make public hospitals autonomous, and fund their services publicly	• Public hospitals can be managed more professionally. • Explicit purchasing of services can make hospitals more accountable and improve performance.	• Without changes in the legal environment and ability to release low-performing workers, savings may not be realized. • Unless social mandates (such as free care for the poor) are made more measurable and sufficient budgets are provided, social mandates and efficiencies may not be realized. • Moral hazard: Because it is unlikely that governments would allow public hospitals to be closed, market exposure of such institutions will be limited. • Professional hospital management has not been well developed in India, so expected management improvements may not be achieved. • Bureaucratic opposition to relinquishing control over hospital administration may make such reforms difficult. • Opposition from labor unions and doctors may be anticipated, particularly if losses of employment or benefits appear possible.

Note: MOHFW, Ministry of Health and Family Welfare.

112

ner in which the poor and the sick will be subsidized; the package of health services to be covered; and the payment mechanisms to be used. The health information systems, clinical networks, and quality assurance procedures that health insurance will depend on will also require considerable effort to develop.

Relying on private health insurance (action 3) is likely to play some role in the short term because the insurance market has been liberalized and its use consumes little in the way of additional public resources. However, it would still be desirable for the central government to play a larger role in actively regulating private insurance, although states could contribute to the monitoring and regulating of health insurance. International experience has shown that the cost of not aggressively regulating private voluntary health insurance is escalating health costs, increased inequalities, and greater difficulty in regulating it later on.

Options for the reform of hospital operations are complementary to those oriented around financing. For states earlier in the transition and with less capacity (category C), governments might reasonably spend more effort on improving the quality of existing public first-referral hospitals but do it in a selective manner that would promote more equitable distribution of public resources (action 4). Experience with projects to develop state health systems has shown that such approaches can improve quality of care and efficiency, although several years of work are required before many of the benefits are seen. Many countries have tried to make the type of changes in hospital organization addressed in action 5, but few have been able to obtain the full set of benefits intended at the start of reforms. Nonetheless, given the degree of inefficiencies and discontent in public hospitals, some states may find it attractive to make hospitals more autonomous in the hope that they can be managed more professionally and made more accountable.

Putting It All Together: The Case of Maternal Health

In the previous section, we examined in broad terms how different states have different priorities and opportunities to make different choices for their future health system. In this section, we take a look at how to put the choices together for a particular program. We use the example of maternal health because it is a national priority, its range of activities span all aspects of the health system, and it illustrates the variety of interrelationships among the pieces of the health system. Below are four visions of how maternal health services could be directed in India. Table 4.10 summarizes how these visions would be implemented for a detailed set of maternal health activities.

Vision 1: A revitalized, vertically integrated, publicly provided system. Vision 1 is for all maternity services to be delivered and financed through the public sector. The public sector would provide the facilities and staff for universal prenatal, delivery, and postnatal care. A benefit of this vision, if realized, is the expansion of opportunities to provide child health and health education services. A large increase in public finances and a change in the way the public service works (especially with respect to staff placement and discipline) would be needed to attract patients from the private sector. Because all service would be rendered free of direct charge to patients, health insurance would not be required.

Vision 2: A private sector system with public financing for the poor and public oversight. In this vision, the private sector would provide all services, and the public sector would provide financing through vouchers of insurance for services provided to the poor or other identified groups. Few savings would be realized from a reduction in staff and capital for prenatal and postnatal care unless all ambulatory care were also privatized. Referral networks to handle complicated cases would need to be strengthened within the private sector, and systems of accrediting quality providers would need to be put in place. Incentive schemes would also be needed to attract private sector and NGO providers to offer services in remote and poor regions. Provider associations could be encouraged to promote safe motherhood.

Table 4.10 Allocation of Critical Health System Functions for Maternal Care between the Public and Private Sectors, by Type of Vision for Public-Private Partnerships

FUNCTION	SPECIFIC COMPONENTS	VISION 1	VISION 2	VISION 3	VISION 4
Oversight	• Health management information systems on access and utilization of services by poor, cesarean delivery rates, etc. • Placement and incentive policies • Quality assurance on clinical standards, cesarean deliveries, blood banks, and training of clinicians	Public sector responsibility for financing and possibly implementation. Private firms or independent agencies may be contracted to design and implement some of these tasks. Goodwill with the private sector needs to be developed to extend coverage to private sector			
Public health services	Behavior change communications on: • Age at marriage • Birth spacing • Early registration for prenatal care • Signs of high-risk pregnancies • Use of referral services	Public sector responsibility for financing and possibly implementation. Private firms may be contracted to design, implement or monitor these tasks.			
Ambulatory care	• Prenatal care (blood pressure measurement, abdominal palpation, blood and urine test, iron folic acid supplements, tetanus toxoid) • Home visits (prenatal and postnatal) • Timely identification of high risk • Referral transport • Mapping of referral facilities	Public implementation and financing	Private implementation Public financing for the poor	Private implementation Private financing or public financing for the poor	Shared implementation Networking between public and private sectors

(Table continues on the following page.)

115

Table 4.10 (continued)

FUNCTION	SPECIFIC COMPONENTS	VISION 1	VISION 2	VISION 3	VISION 4
Inpatient care	• Prenatal complications • Delivery (normal and assisted) • Emergency obstetric care • Blood transfusion • Care of newborn (normal and sick) • Postnatal complications	Public implementation	Private implementation Public financing for the poor (vouchers or insurance)	Shared, public funding of public hospitals	Shared implementation Public insurance for poor or single payer for all
Financing	• Payment (out-of-pocket; free care; insurance	Public financing	Shared (public funds focused on the poor)	Shared (public funds focused on poor)	Shared (public funds used for poor, or for those with complications, or for all)

Note: For definitions of visions, see text.

Vision 3: Public sector health promotion, private sector prenatal visits and routine deliveries, and public sector emergency care. In this vision, the public sector focuses on advancing awareness of good health practices such as sufficient birth intervals, the use of prenatal care and safe abortions, and institutional deliveries; the implementation of communication programs may be done through private sector agencies. Prenatal care and routine deliveries would be done primarily through the private sector and emergency obstetric care primarily through public sector hospitals.

Vision 4: Public sector health promotion, private and public prenatal care, insurance for institutional deliveries in either public or private sector. In this vision, the public sector would again be responsible for the promotive health communications. The current mix of public and private prenatal care would continue or could be enhanced through quality assurance procedures and networking that would involve both public and private providers. Insurance could cover the higher costs of institutional deliveries and any complications through a number of approaches, such as (a) voluntary insurance with public insurance for the poor, (b) mandated private purchase of insurance policies of choice and public financing of insurance for the poor, and (c) publicly funded single payer insurance. Emergency obstetric care could be provided through either public or private hospitals, and financed through insurance.

The implementation of any one of these four visions for maternal services would have its own set of challenges and risks. Vision 1 may fit best with the traditional rhetoric of the health system. However, the private sector is currently providing large portions of the ambulatory and inpatient care for maternity services. In the absence of considerable increases or shifts in public spending and a feasible plan to replace the private sector, vision 1 may be the least realistic of the four visions. Vision 2 may be the most politically difficult of the four because it envisions the largest reduction in the public sector's direct delivery of services.

Visions 3 and 4 rely more on shared approaches; they have the advantages of being susceptible to implementation in steps and of using the private sector while giving greater attention to the needs of the poor. However, vision 3 would entail a difficult and at times arbitrary reduction in public services for prenatal and routine deliveries while requiring the public sector to expand its emergency care. Opposition from the labor force and politicians could be expected, and efficiency gains in the public sector are hard to imagine if it must maintain and expand its emergency obstetric services. Vision 4 takes most advantage of the current situation and may offer less political resistance, although it depends on the development of meaningful partnerships between public and private sectors that have so far eluded the health system. It also depends on insurance schemes that have yet to be tested on a significant scale.

Specific Actions for Consideration across India

Up to this point, we have assessed options without prescribing specific recommendations for the reform of India's health sector. In this section we advance such concrete proposals. The intention is not to prescribe detailed steps but to further the discussion and decision-making about India's health system. These proposals for translating the options into policy and action are offered in that spirit.

Health Policy

National health policy, last articulated in the 1983 Health Policy and the National Population Policy (Ministry of Health and Family Welfare 2000b), is being revised and preparations are being made for the 10th Five-Year Plan as this is written. We argue that in the updating of its policies and plans, India must give more attention than it has in the past to the monitoring of health system outcomes and to improving the distribution of services among different groups of Indians, particularly the poor. Given the great variation in conditions among the states, revisions in national policy also ought to allow greater specificity and flexibility in dealing with the various states. In particular, the new plans must discover ways that national priority programs can be productively decentralized to states and local bodies and ways that the central government can provide relevant support to states facing different issues. The questions raised in this chapter about central government allocations to health should also be clarified.

Shortcomings in policy are even greater at the state level. No state has a comprehensive policy or strategy for dealing with the health sector. All of them should have plans that encompass the issues confronting the national government, but in addition, the states ought to address how they intend to integrate centrally sponsored schemes and state health programs and how they can be monitored. Thus, both the national and state-level plans must be sensitive to the existence of the other.

The studies supporting this report make it clear that national and state health policies must take a far more comprehensive and operational approach to dealing with the private sector if these policies hope to accomplish the following:

- Improve the quality of services in the private sector and build systems to assure quality (for example, accreditation systems, focused regulations, and public disclosure)

- Reduce inequity in charges in the private sector and build transparency in the pricing of private health services (for example, through publicly disclosed pricing guidelines)

- Define the rights and obligations of the public with respect to health services provided by the private health sector (for example, a charter of patient rights)

- Outline the requirements for sharing of information with the private sector (for example, on clinical care, outcomes, and costs)

- Create tools to control costs and encourage appropriate utilization in the private sector (for example, mandatory review for high-cost procedures and hospitalizations)

- Define what government agencies will offer to private providers under service agreements (for example, information, materials, immunizations, and drugs for national programs such as tuberculosis)

- Find opportunities to increase access to health services through the private sector (for example, through joint ventures, incentives for service in remote areas)

- Determine what types of subsidies will support public policy objectives (for example, land in rural areas for clinics)

- Lay ground rules for public-private partnerships in health services (for example, by contracting and by extending provider networks and referral systems to the private sector)

- Develop strategies for dealing with practitioners without medical qualifications

- Place boundaries on the roles of various types of organizational structures in the health sector (for example, public oversight boards, large inpatient facilities, for-profit corporations, and local bodies).

Operational Steps

In addition to articulating health policies that would deal with these neglected areas of the health system, it is also important to find means to translate them into action. Without repeating the rationale for each of the various options discussed in the preceding chapter, we now propose a number of important options that can be taken up by government (table 4.11). Steps to be taken in the near to medium term are the more feasible or are prerequisites to larger reforms. For example, experimentation in health financing and the development of health information systems and quality assurance are proposed as steps that need to be taken before establishing a long-term health financing system. The proposals outlined are also selected because they allow the government to follow a particular vision it may develop for the sector, thereby leaving open as many options as possible.

Table 4.11 Recommendations for Government Action on Critical Functions of India's Health System

FUNCTION	SHORT- AND MEDIUM-TERM MEASURES	LONG-TERM MEASURES
Health system oversight	• Update national health policy and specify roles for private sector • Develop state health policies • Invest in drug quality control • Invest in disease surveillance and control • Invest in health and management information systems for public and private sector • Monitor distribution and levels of public utilization and subsidies • Expand and share knowledge base about health system performance • Establish public-private forums on health care • Develop human resource development plans at national and state levels, including new capacities	• Evaluate private and public provider performance • Publicly disclose pricing of health services • Accredit hospitals based on quality • License or relicense health providers • Implement human resource development plan • Revise mechanisms for consumer redress in health care
Public health services	• In early health transition states, focus on injuries, and improved implementation and decentralization of centrally sponsored schemes • Expand health promotion of unfinished agenda and HIV control • Provide public information on health service performance and rights of public	• Expand public health programs for tobacco control, mental health (short- to medium-term action in some states)
Ambulatory curative care	• Eliminate inpatient beds at public primary health centers • Begin measuring quality, costs, efficiency, and social mandates in private and public sectors • Experiment with greater contracting of services with NGOs and private sector	• Promote mixed public-private provision through greater networking, contracting, and shared training and information and with clear public accountabilities • Promote greater specialization and professional management of public sector logistic support systems

(Table continues on the following page.)

Table 4.11 (continued)

FUNCTION	SHORT- AND MEDIUM-TERM MEASURES	LONG-TERM MEASURES
	• Invest on improving quality rather than expansion of publicly provided services • If no increase in public financing, pay for oversight and public health activities through reductions in public funding of ambulatory curative care	(e.g., drug and equipment procurement and management) for minor and inpatient care • Separate health providers from civil service (for both out-patient and inpatient care)
Inpatient care	• Rationalize services and develop dynamic need and performance-based service norms at state level • Develop policy and plans for dealing with long-term inpatient stays, currently dominated by the rich • Improve measurability of quality, costs, efficiency, and social mandates in private and public sectors • Experiment with increased autonomy of public hospitals • Develop service agreements with hospitals run by NGOs and by private firms • If no increase in funds, limit public spending at tertiary hospitals and focus resources on fewer tertiary institutions and rural secondary hospitals	• Promote mixed public-private provision through greater networking, contracting, and shared training and information and with clear public accountabilities • Decentralize local management of public and private hospitals through local governments and public boards
Health financing	• Experiment with prepayment risk pooling of sufficient scale (e.g., at least one district) • Actively regulate private, voluntary health insurance (see chapter 7 for details)	• Establish publicly accountable administration of health insurance with universal coverage (single payer or multiple plans) • Increase revenues for health through general taxation and special taxes on health-harming products (e.g., tobacco and alcohol).

122

These recommendations are supported by the four principles advanced at the outset of this chapter for raising the sights of India's health system:

1. Oversee the needs of the whole population

2. Look forward to new challenges of the health system

3. Remove a large blind spot by making better use of the private sector

4. Focus on improving quality, efficiency, and accountability of health services.

The initial steps include measures to broaden the scope of the health policy framework while making it more operational, increase "measurability" in the health sector, add more experimentation and flexibility in approaches, and rely more extensively on public-private partnerships.

An Agenda for the Future

As India's health system continues to evolve, an ongoing process of analysis, discussion, and informed decision is needed to meet the challenges. The need to better understand the main actors, functions, and outcomes of the health system will continue. And the wide variation in conditions across India demand that local investigation be carried out so that solutions can be custom-made to particular states and districts.

If India's health system is to address the needs of the entire population in an effective, efficient, and accountable manner, people from all segments of society must become engaged in decisions about the future direction of the health system, and the health system must find ways of facilitating such broad engagement. If India is to face the challenge of the health transition, then different approaches to health financing and new public health programs will be needed. If India is to take advantage of all its resources in the health sector, the energies of the private sector need to be harnessed and market failures counteracted. The public sector will also need to better oversee the health sector on behalf of all citizens, especially the poor and the vulnerable.

Important gaps still remain in our knowledge about and experience in the Indian health system. Appendix table 4A.1 outlines these gaps and indicates how the information filling those gaps could be applied. Here are some of the most pressing areas for more detailed analysis and consideration of options:

- Working effectively with the informal sector of private health providers within the boundaries defined by law.

- Testing new health financing systems.

- Analyzing pharmaceutical policy in the context of a new international trade regime and the challenge of emerging diseases. In particular, examining how HIV drugs can be made affordable in India.

- Analyzing options for urban health care.

- Testing innovative approaches to delivering services for the unfinished agenda, particularly neonatal health and malnutrition.

- Developing strategies for health manpower development, in particular how to strengthen public health and nursing capacity, and how to reform medical education.

- Understanding how to maximize the benefits from health research and development.

Concluding Remarks

This report began by observing that India's health system is at a crossroads. The study process generated a considerable amount of new information about the workings of the Indian health system and revealed many options for reform; it also showed that no single choice or path is best for all of India. Particular conditions and particular states require their own mixes of policy and timing. So those seeking new approaches must travel with eyes open, consciously deciding which fork in the road to take for each situation. Discovering the right way requires experimentation, consultation, analysis, debate, and the forging of a consensus on key issues.

Now is the time to conduct big experiments in India's health sector, particularly since the status quo is leading to a dead end. Either the national government or individual states could take the initiative, but new experience is needed to build on what has become an outmoded health system. The opportunity exists now for governments to reform the way they work and take on critical oversight functions. Governments also need to consider new ways to implement new and existing public health services. New ways of managing ambulatory and inpatient services should also be tried, along with a concerted effort to develop a more efficient, equitable, and risk-reducing health financing system. The new experiments need to build in flexibility to deal with very different conditions in India and to provide a basis for learning through intensive monitoring and evaluation. In the long run, this approach will better enable India to meet the health needs of its people.

Appendix

Table 4A.1 Key Gaps in Knowledge about and Experience in India's Health System, and Potential Uses of the Needed Information

GAPS IN KNOWLEDGE AND EXPERIENCE	USE OF INFORMATION
Role of the public	
• How to empower people to better manage their health	• Improved programs to strengthen people's ability to manage their health
Role of public and private sectors	
• Understanding the constraints, means of operation, and performance of the private sector in health in local markets	• Design and implement interventions to influence the effectiveness and equity of the private sector in health, and improve accountability
• Feasibility of health networks involving NGO and private providers	• Models for providing comprehensive health care to more people
• Evaluation of contracting mechanisms in health	• Appropriate expansion of good management practices
Financing functions	
• Feasibility of health insurance schemes (social insurance, community prepayment)	• Working model of health insurance or community financing schemes
• Unit costs for health services provided in different settings	• Means to improve the efficiency of health services, and better negotiate with private sector
• Analysis of alternative financing schemes for NGOs—feasibility studies	• Mechanisms to improve selection and performance of health NGOs
Input management	
• How to prepare for the new TRIPS regime in pharmaceuticals. How to develop, finance, and make available affordable drugs for HIV and other emerging conditions	• Plans for making new pharmaceuticals affordable and available in India
• How to reorganize and strengthen health manpower, particularly in key areas of public health, nursing, management	• Renewed education and training programs for key health professions

Service delivery

- Innovative approaches to addressing the "unfinished agenda"
- How to reorganize public hospitals

- How well can responsibilities in the public health sector be decentralized
- How to work effectively with untrained medical practitioners

- How to take successful but small community health programs to scale
- How to appropriately integrate various health programs at state and local levels

Health systems outcomes

- Obtaining data through special surveys and building systems to collect and use information on cause of death, financial impact of illness and health services, and satisfaction with health services, with special focus on vulnerable groups

- More effective and locally responsive priority programs
- New ways to improve the efficiency, accountability, and social mandates of public hospitals
- How to strengthen capacity of states and local bodies in health delivery, including options for integrating health programs
- Find ways to eliminate harmful practices and to use untrained practitioners to extend health services in underserved areas
- Scaling up of useful public health programs.

- More efficient and effective health services

- Better monitoring, evaluation, and planning of health resources and services

Note: TRIPS, trade-related aspects of intellectual property.

Notes

1. Higher use of hospitalization does not necessarily imply that people are sicker. Chapter 2 (table 2.2) showed that levels of hospitalization and outpatient visits are lower in India than in other low-income countries. Rates of inpatient and outpatient use were progressively higher in higher-income countries.

2. These classifications are somewhat arbitrary; they are intended to be only indicative, partly because state capacity is not directly measured. Full immunization coverage rates were used as an indicator of public service capacity since these are largely delivered through the public sector.

3. Adding the state private sector hospitalization rate changes the rank order of some of the states, but they cluster within the same four categories of states.

4. But this may also indicate the existence of a two-tier delivery system in which the poor rely on the public sector and the better-off use the private sector.

5. As noted later in this chapter, this is still a simplification of the type of choices faced by these states. Institutional deliveries and first-referral hospital care for diseases such as pneumonia and tuberculosis are critical to the success of these public programs.

6. National Sample Survey rates are based on self-reported regular use and are not adjusted for differences in the age structures of state populations.

7. These recommendations include: merging of the Departments of Health, Family Welfare, and Indian Systems of Medicine; full autonomization of institutions of national importance and the Central Government Health Scheme (CGHS); handing over the admin-

istration of hospital facilities in the capital region to the Delhi government; devolving responsibility for most of the 19 centrally sponsored schemes to the states; establishing an independent organization to ensure medical education standards; developing more operational policies for working with the private sector; and completely restructuring the Directorate General of Health Services to become a health policy and technical support organization for health information and monitoring, thereby terminating its duties as an administrator of health services, purchaser of drugs and supplies, and executive of drug quality control.

8. The states are Andhra Pradesh, Karnataka, Maharashtra, Orissa, Punjab, Uttar Pradesh, and West Bengal.

9. Several reasons exist for the central government to spend more on health services in states experiencing civil conflict, but this report does not assess options particular to conditions of civil conflict.

PART 2

Theory and Evidence

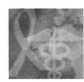

CHAPTER 5

Health System Framework

Health status is widely recognized as both an input and an outcome of broader social and economic developments. As an outcome, health gains arise out of improvements in the general standard of living rather than simply from improvements in the health sector alone.[1] As an input, good health improves educational attainment and fosters economic growth and political participation. By the same token, ill health and poor health services are increasingly recognized as major causes of poverty, so efforts to combat poverty ought to consider the role of health (box 5.1).

In describing health systems, the international literature tends to focus on institutions and services whose primary purpose is to protect and improve health.[2] Other factors that influence health are usually considered as part of the health system's external environment, that is, outside its boundaries. Even though such an approach inevitably involves some ambiguous or arbitrary distinctions (for example, deworming of children may be part of a school program rather than a health service), defining these boundaries is still useful in conceptualizing a health system and in examining the choices that are possible for its development.

More specifically, here is our approach to the description of India's health system and to the analysis of how to improve it:

- We adapt a model used in the *World Health Report 2000* (WHO 2000c) to describe the actors, functions, and outcomes of a health system.

- To assess *whether* government should finance or provide certain health services, we use an economic framework that relies both on traditional public economics and a concern for equity.

- To address the more difficult questions of *the extent* to which government should intervene and the extent to which markets should play a role, we utilize a framework borrowed from the field of institutional economics. That framework clarifies the areas in which direct government production is needed and those in which other choices should be made for financing or contracting for goods and services.

- We also recognize that policymaking is not a linear process, that choices of action are determined by social and political preferences, and that such preferences are influenced by the experiences and interests and values of different groups.

Box 5.1 How Chronic Illness Makes People Poor

Poor people see good health as a major asset. Illness is disabling and costly, especially when a breadwinner or other active adult is struck down. A commonly encountered scenario starts with illness or injury causing an immediate loss of income from work. The afflicted person either goes without treatment, or treatment is received but the costs impoverish the family. Assets are sold and debts taken on. Thus begins a downward spiral from which the family may never recover. Food becomes scarce. Children may become malnourished, and they are withdrawn from school to save money and to work. The poor household becomes permanently poorer. When an active adult dies, the ratio of dependants to adults jumps up. The problem worsens when an active adult becomes permanently disabled: the person can no longer work but must still be fed.

A case in point is the family of Padma, a 30-year-old woman who lives in Geruwa, a village on the outskirts of Tatanagar in south Bihar. She has four daughters, the eldest of whom is seven years old. Padma's husband used to work in a dairy, cleaning buffaloes, but he suffers from diabetes and can no longer do labor-intensive work.

To raise money for her husband's ongoing treatment, Padma sold her house and land to another resident of the village for Rs 1,300, although the actual value was more than Rs 20,000. She knows she was underpaid but feels indebted to the buyer because he has allowed her to use a small room in the house to shelter her children and ailing husband. The daughters do not go to school, and she is reluctant for them to do so. Padma has taken over the support of the family by carrying wood fuel on her head for a distance of about 10 kilometers every other day. She and her family live hand to mouth, as her earnings are just enough to purchase 2 kilograms of rice a day.

Source: Narayan and others (2000).

The Descriptive Framework: Health System Actors, Functions, and Outcomes

Three elements constitute our description of the health system: actors (people and institutions), functions (the things they do), and outcomes (the results of what they do).

Actors

In our simplified framework of the health system (figure 5.1), we examine three broad categories of actors: people, the state, and private sector actors.

- People are placed at the top of the health system because we consider the promotion, maintenance, and recovery of people's health to be the defining characteristics of a health system.

- The state is represented by the ministries and departments of health and family welfare at central, state, and local levels, government entities whose primary activities are most closely related to the health sector. Other important public bodies that affect the health system include the judiciary, the ministry of finance, planning commissions, and sectoral ministries such as those for women and child development, education, and water and sanitation.

- Private sector actors include both for-profit and nonprofit health providers, practitioners of allopathic (or Western) and other systems of medicine, and untrained, informal providers. Beyond the private health providers are the private sector actors involved in financing of health care and in the management of other inputs to the health sector.

The health system also responds to demand, which is created by people. Demand for health services in turn creates the main health sector market—a point worth emphasizing. The health sector encompasses many types of ancillary markets as well—for example the markets for pharmaceuticals, medical manpower, and diagnostics, and these markets do not necessarily compete with each other. These markets are part of the context for the functions of the health system.

Functions

In our framework, the functions of the health system (shown in the ovals in figure 5.1) are financing, management of nonfinancial inputs, health service delivery itself, and oversight.[3]

Responsibilities for the first three sets of functions considered—financing, management of inputs, and service delivery—are currently shared between private sector and public actors.

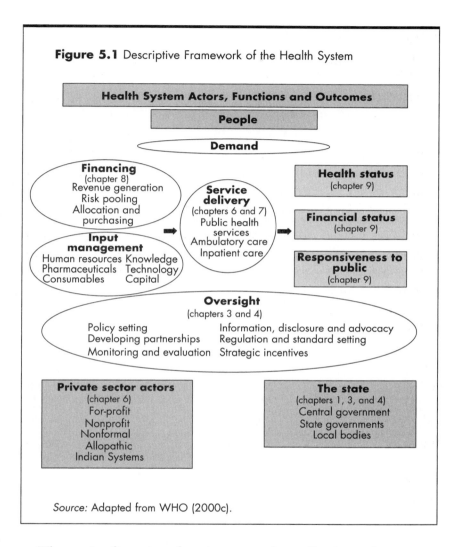

Figure 5.1 Descriptive Framework of the Health System

Health System Actors, Functions and Outcomes

People

Demand

Financing
(chapter 8)
Revenue generation
Risk pooling
Allocation and
purchasing

Input management
Human resources Knowledge
Pharmaceuticals Technology
Consumables Capital

Service delivery
(chapters 6 and 7)
Public health
services
Ambulatory care
Inpatient care

Health status
(chapter 9)

Financial status
(chapter 9)

Responsiveness to public
(chapter 9)

Oversight
(chapters 3 and 4)

Policy setting   Information, disclosure and advocacy
Developing partnerships   Regulation and standard setting
Monitoring and evaluation Strategic incentives

Private sector actors
(chapter 6)
For-profit
Nonprofit
Nonformal
Allopathic
Indian Systems

The state
(chapters 1, 3, and 4)
Central government
State governments
Local bodies

Source: Adapted from WHO (2000c).

The main financing functions are the collection of revenues through taxes and insurance premiums, the pooling of funds through insurance, and the allocation of revenues through purchase of services or budget transfers to health providers.

The management of nonfinancial inputs is the gathering and use of assets such as human resources, knowledge and software, drugs, physical capital such as medical equipment and buildings, and supplies.

Service delivery functions are divided among public health services, ambulatory clinical services, and inpatient, hospital-based, clinical services. The nature of the services may be preventive, diagnostic, therapeutic, rehabilitative, or palliative.

The fourth main function, oversight, is largely a responsibility of the state. The concept of oversight goes beyond the conventional idea of regulation—setting and enforcing rules—to other functions such as developing policy and providing strategic direction to the health system. Oversight may also require mediation between different actors in the health sector to set a level playing field (negotiating between health providers or financiers) or facilitating the improvement of performance (such as promoting or mandating professional self-regulation). Other oversight roles are the development of partnerships or networks among health service providers and financiers and the strategic use of incentives to promote public policy objectives.

Acquiring and disseminating information about performance, quality, or pricing is another oversight function, one intended to guide the health-related decisions of the public, policymakers, and providers. Even if government does not undertake the monitoring and evaluation itself, it has a primary interest in ensuring that monitoring and evaluation occurs and that the information is used for policy and implementation responses. Examples of nongovernmental bodies providing oversight functions are consumer organizations disclosing good medical practice and professional bodies engaging in self-regulation.

The distinctions made between some of these functions may be somewhat arbitrary because the functions are often closely related. People's demand for, say, healthy deliveries, creates markets for more particular services (fetal ultrasound testing, for example) and products (perhaps new drugs). Oversight activities influence each of the other actors and functions. The management of inputs is tied to the types of services delivered; how they are paid for affects their quality, quantity, and distribution.

Public health is also divided among several functions. In its basic definition, public health involves the programs and institutions organized by society to protect, promote, and restore people's health. By its nature, public health involves the maintenance and improvement of health through collective or social actions. These public health functions are largely divided into oversight activities and the public health programs. The oversight functions are primarily directed at private sector and government actors on behalf of the citizenry. Public health programs are aimed directly at the public, either as individuals, communities, or larger populations. In some cases, such as the control of tuberculosis and malaria, public health services also overlap with ambulatory care and hospital services.

Outcomes

The health system has three types of outcomes (boxes on the right side of figure 5.1): health status, financial status, and consumer responsiveness.[4] The outcomes begin with traditional measures of health status, such as rates for mortality, nutrition, fertility, illness, and disability, which are the most important considerations of a health system. For the sake of simplicity, figure 5.1 does not include the important underlying determinants of health outcomes that fall outside the health sector, such as education, income, and use of sanitation facilities and safe water.

The second health system outcome, financial status, is a measure of the financial loss due to illness, which can include direct costs of health care and earnings lost because of illness. The concern is not only about how costs affect equity in access, but also the risk of loss of income and assets. Financial protection is particularly important to the poor, as the costs of ill health push people into poverty and deepen the levels of poverty.

Consumer responsiveness of the health system is measured by how satisfied the public is with various aspects of health services. It also includes consideration of whether health services treat people with respect and whether they are provided with protection against malpractice and exploitation.[5] Here again, the poor are just as concerned with dignity and with being treated respectfully by the health system as are those who are wealthier and more powerful.

How can India's health system meet its fundamental objectives in an equitable, effective, accountable, and affordable manner? This question, which is also considered in the analysis, raises a second order of objectives relevant for the health system, though not shown in figure 5.1. This level of intermediate objectives may include the following parameters: [6]

- *Equity*. Some minimum of health care should be accessible to all citizens in accordance with their needs, at least in services publicly financed. Equity can also be considered in other terms, such as an equal distribution of public expenditure on health, equal use of health services, or equal health outcomes.

- *Efficiency and quality*. Health services should provide the optimum combination of good outcomes—good health, financial protection, and consumer satisfaction (allocative efficiency), with costs minimized for a given output (cost and technical efficiency). Another way of stating this is that quality of health services should be optimized, which can be considered in terms of technical quality of services (how well the interventions provided work), managerial quality (how well outputs are maximized given the level of inputs), and perception of quality (how well patients are satisfied with services).

- *Macroeconomic efficiency*. Health expenditure should consume an appropriate proportion of GDP.

- *Consumer choice*. The public should have a sufficient choice of providers in both public and private sectors.

- *Provider autonomy*. Doctors and health providers should have the maximum freedom compatible with the attainment of other health system objectives.

The overall levels of health system outcomes are important, but so too is the distribution of the results among different geographic

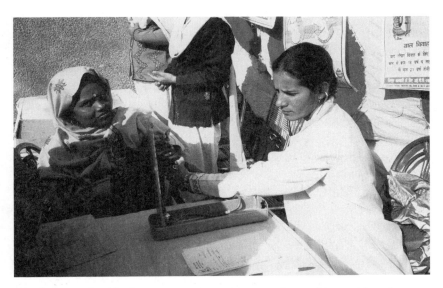

Checkup at a health clinic (PHOTOGRAPH BY GEETANJALI CHOPRA/HEMANT MEHTA/ THE WORLD BANK)

areas and populations, and particularly for various vulnerable groups such as the poor, scheduled castes and tribes, women, and the young. Distributional aspects are examined in detail in this report. Although health status is the most important health outcome, we also argue that all three health system objectives are important in India and should be addressed systematically with an eye to the implications for the poor.

As we discuss later in this report, some of these objectives can be pursued at little cost and do not necessarily take away resources from activities that directly affect health status. This report examines why the health transition that is occurring in India lends urgency to the reform of India's health system financing and to making it more responsive. Dealing with financing and consumer responsiveness can also contribute to the improvement of targeted health outcomes through gains in quality, access, accountability, and efficiency of health services.

Framework for the Consideration of Government Intervention

The descriptive framework outlined above provides a good basis for understanding the various health system functions and for orienting its key actors toward a fundamental set of objectives. To fully assess the options for government intervention, we need to build on this understanding so we can delve further into the alternatives and the question of how to choose among them.

A first-level question is whether the public sector should intervene in the health sector. Public economics theory provides one set of answers to this question. The basic rationales for intervention are to: (a) ensure provision of public goods or services with large externalities,[7] (b) provide a safety net to alleviate poverty, and (c) correct for market failure, either when access to appropriate health services is limited or when the insurance market has failed. The studies included in this report help to clarify these choices by showing how the poor are affected by health services, identifying the beneficiaries of public sector services, and spotlighting areas in which the private market is failing.

Figure 5.2 shows decision points for government intervention that are based on a combination of traditional public economics (public goods, externalities, demand, catastrophic costs) and a concern for equity. This chart makes clear that while the health system may have one set of objectives, the various activities in the health system are not fungible or homogeneous goods and services. If one is concerned with "public health" services that are not individualized curative care services, then the decision process is much different from that if the concern is for curative care. Within curative care, we distinguish services involving "catastrophic" cost, a level of expense we used above to distinguish between ambulatory and inpatient care.[8]

Public finance economics provides a robust justification for public oversight of the health system (regulation of private providers and health insurance), for public financing of health services when large externalities exist (communicable disease control, reproductive health programs, health promotion, training), and for targeted pub-

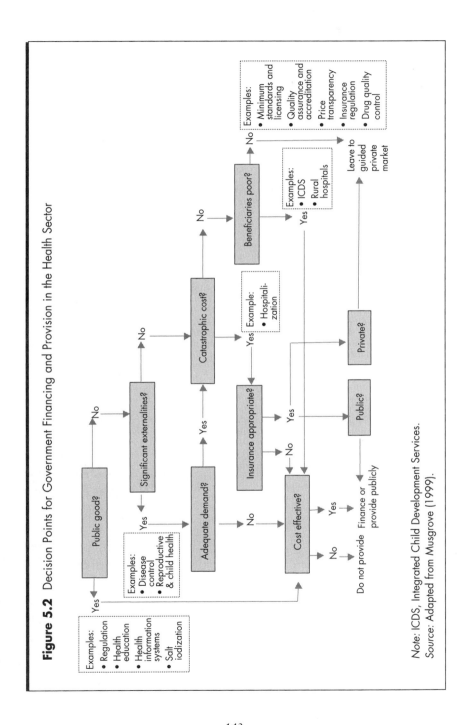

Figure 5.2 Decision Points for Government Financing and Provision in the Health Sector

Public good?

Examples:
• Regulation
• Health education
• Health information systems
• Salt iodization

Significant externalities?

Examples:
• Disease control
• Reproductive & child health

Adequate demand?

Catastrophic cost?

Beneficiaries poor?

Examples:
• Minimum standards and licensing
• Quality assurance and accreditation
• Price transparency
• Insurance regulation
• Drug quality control

Examples:
• ICDS
• Rural hospitals

Example:
• Hospitalization

Insurance appropriate?

Cost effective?

Private?

Public?

leave to guided private market

Finance or provide publicly

Do not provide

Yes / No

Note: ICDS, Integrated Child Development Services.
Source: Adapted from Musgrove (1999).

143

lic programs for the poor (rural health facilities, financing fee exemptions for the poor). However, this approach also has its limitations: that is, one must account for historical context, social preferences, and political processes and also move beyond the question of *whether* government should intervene to the question of *how* government should intervene.

A Framework for Deciding How to Intervene: Make-Buy-Regulate-Inform

A useful new framework for looking at how government can intervene in the health sector takes advantage of tools of institutional economics (Girishankar 1999; Preker, Harding, and Travis 2000). Using two basic characteristics of goods and services, contestability and measurability, the framework lays out the market conditions for the inputs (factors of production) as well as the services (products) in the health sector.

Contestability is the extent to which a market can be entered and exited freely. Markets that are highly contestable have low barriers to entry by new providers and mechanisms (such as bankruptcy protection) that allow the easy exit of existing providers. Markets that have low contestability have high barriers to entry by new providers because, for example, entry requires large sunk costs or existing providers wield monopoly power or have geographic advantages. Measurability is the extent to which it is easy to measure important elements such as inputs, processes, outputs, and outcomes.

The framework allows policymakers to examine different aspects of the health sector and assess the degree to which direct government provision may be necessary ("make") and the conditions under which purchasing may be used instead ("buy"). Figures 5.3 and 5.4 give examples of the application of this framework. Figure 5.3 shows that the difficulty of measuring health outputs explains where difficulties may lie in dealing with the product markets of health service delivery. Measurement issues also help explain why contracting out for laundry and catering services, whose outputs are quite measura-

Figure 5.3 Measurability and Contestability of Health Services
(Product Markets)

		Contestability		
		High	Medium	Low
Measurability	High	Type I	Type II	Type III
	Medium	Type IV • Nonclinical activities – Management support – Laundry & catering • Routine diagnostics	Type V • Clinical interventions • High-tech diagnostics	Type VI • Monitoring/evaluation
	Low	Type VII • Ambulatory care – Medical – Nursing – Dental	Type VIII • Public health interventions • Intersectoral action • Inpatient care	Type IX • Policymaking

Source: Preker, Harding, and Travis (2000).

ble and whose markets are highly contestable, makes more sense than contracting out for ambulatory care, whose market may be highly contestable but whose outputs are very difficult to measure. The situation in the factor market, which comprises the inputs to the health system, is quite different. Figure 5.4 shows that its measurability in factor markets is less of an issue than for services but that contestability for the factor markets is more important than it is for services markets.

This framework can be used not only to outline the nature of goods and services in the health sector but also to identify policy levers to improve the functioning of the markets. Figure 5.5 indicates that buying services is a more feasible option when measurability is high, and buying inputs is more feasible when contestability is high.

Figure 5.4 Measurability and Contestability of Inputs (Factor Markets) in the Health Sector

		Contestability		
		High	Medium	Low

Measurability	High	Type I
		• Production of consumables
		• Retail of
		  – Drugs & equipment
		  – Other consumables
		• Unskilled labor
			Type II
			• Production of equipment
			• Wholesale
			  – Drugs & equipment
			  – Other consumables
			• Small capital stock
				Type III
				• Production
				  – Pharmaceuticals
				  – High technology
				• Large capital stock

	Medium	Type IV	Type V
			• Basic training
			  – Skilled labor
				Type VI
				• Research
				  – Knowledge
				• Higher education
				  – High-skilled labor

	Low	Type VII	Type VIII	Type IX

Source: Preker, Harding, and Travis (2000)

Figure 5.5 also shows how various policy tools can improve the functioning of the markets. Disclosing data concerning quality, prices, and effectiveness of health services increases both measurability and contestability. In some cases, the availability of such information makes market provision of goods and services more feasible or improves the potential for government to purchase services.

Policies that increase the availability of information, enable health providers and organizations to use such information, and increase patients' understanding of illness and health services have positive effects on contestability and measurability in the health system. Monetization of social benefits, such as measuring and financing services provided to the poor, can also help improve contestability and ensure that these benefits are provided in both public and pri-

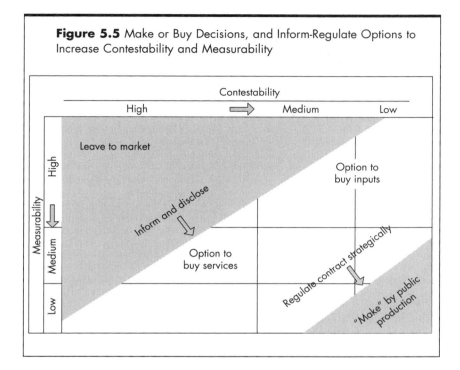

Figure 5.5 Make or Buy Decisions, and Inform-Regulate Options to Increase Contestability and Measurability

vate sectors. Regulation can be used to increase measurability by changing reporting requirements and accountability mechanisms. Regulation can also be used to reduce barriers to entering the market, such as by reducing the use of noncompetitive bidding to purchase equipment and drugs or by blocking inappropriate political interference in public production and purchasing. Contracts can also be designed to use quantifiable results to trigger performance-related payments.

Other factors besides measurability and contestability are important in understanding how markets in the health sector work, how to level the playing field for public and private providers, and how to get the most out of public and private sector production. Motivation and incentives of providers, financiers, and patients are important;

so are transaction costs, innovation, and experience with regulation and various types of partnerships. In the analysis of the private sector (chapter 6), these factors are examined in detail; they are used to understand the advantages and disadvantages of various arrangements and to provide an empirical basis for choosing options rooted in the Indian experience.

Notes

1. This relationship has been described in the *Poverty Reduction Strategy Sourcebook* (World Bank 2000b).

2. Some of widely used descriptions of health systems and health system reform are found in Roemer (1991), OECD (1992), Frenk (1994), Cassels (1995), and Berman (1995).

3. The four critical activities on which we focus our proposals for action (chapter 1)—delivery of public health services, delivery of ambulatory care services, delivery and financing of inpatient care, and oversight—can be seen as largely overlapping these functions.

4. In chapter 1, we described the objectives of the health system in terms of making progress against these three types of outcomes.

5. The concept of responsiveness used in this report is somewhat different than the definition used in the *World Health Report 2000* (WHO 2000c). That report refers to nonmedical aspects of care and excludes satisfaction per se, which includes medical aspects. We also include legal protection and redress, which were not considered in that report's framework.

6. These are adapted from Barr (1990).

7. In this context, an externality is a benefit that accrues to others (who do not pay for it) when an individual pays for and receives a service or good. Under such circumstances, private entities may not provide as much of the good or service as would be socially beneficial.

8. Even though several of the decision paths flow through a consideration of "cost-effectiveness," activities coming from different paths should not be compared head-to-head. That is, one should not compare a "public health" intervention with a "catastrophic cost" intervention using a cost-effectiveness ratio. Particular programs must be considered only within sets of items that are reasonably comparable (for example, public health campaigns for different diseases).

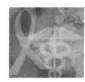

CHAPTER 6

The Functioning of the Private Sector Market

In this chapter, we use new tools of inquiry to examine the characteristics and performance of private health care, and we use Andhra Pradesh and Uttar Pradesh as the "laboratory" for our inquiry (see box 6.1). The object of our attention will be two private health services that, for the most part, do not compete with each other: Ambulatory (outpatient) care and inpatient (hospital-based) care. Product markets, such as those for diagnostic services, are not examined here, nor are factor markets, such as those for pharmaceuticals, medical equipment, private medical colleges, and other suppliers of technology and capital.

Using the theoretical model described in the preceding chapter, we organize the analysis of the private market around three considerations:

- Contestability

- Measurability

- Interactions with the public sector.

To explore contestability, we concentrate on factors that affect the ease of entering or exiting the marketplace. In the cases of ambulatory and inpatient care such factors include reasons for setting up a practice and the manner in which it is set up, including the organizational form chosen for the practice. Access to credit,

Box 6.1 Empirical Findings and Policy Challenges

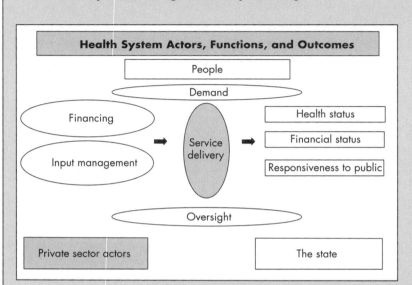

Empirical Findings

- Private health markets differ significantly from state to state. In the two states studied—Andhra Pradesh and Uttar Pradesh—differences were found among private practitioners in the types of cases they see as well as in their therapies, consultation charges, incomes, costs of doing business, concessions offered to the poor, and interest and participation in national health programs.
- Alternative private providers (untrained allopathic doctors and practitioners of nonallopathic medicine) make up the largest segment of the private health care market. Most clinics run by these providers lack expensive equipment, such as microscopes and operating theaters, but are equipped with basic tools, such as thermometers, stethoscopes, and blood pressure gauges.

- Problems with measurability of private sector performance are large, limiting the ability of the private sector to meet health sector objectives. Constraints to entering the market and transaction costs for conducting business are greater for inpatient facilities than for outpatient facilities but are smaller than issues of measurability.
- Irrespective of type of provider, quality assurance in staffing and clinical practice is a problem.
- Although the factors that motivate health workers in the public and private sectors are similar, important differences exist in motivating factors on the job. Public sector workers perceive the lack of training opportunities and the presence of corruption as drawbacks.
- Nearly all private facilities (98 percent) report making concessions to the poor, but they do not document the activity.
- Private sector providers received significantly higher ratings from patients regarding quality and satisfaction than did public sector providers.
- Access to private sources of credit for starting and running new service facilities is relatively easy, and few private hospitals took advantage of public subsidies or exemptions.
- Most private hospitals face problems with public infrastructure such as electricity and drainage, particularly in Uttar Pradesh.

Policy Challenges
- How can public and private health facilities be made more responsive to the needs of their clients? Can client perceptions of providers' manners and skills be incorporated into training and supervision programs to reverse poor treatment?

Box 6.1 (continued)

- What steps can government take to improve performance of the private sector? What are the most effective
  ways of introducing quality assurance systems? Can government create a positive environment for the private
  sector, as opposed to creating an inspectorate raj?
- Can government effectively purchase services from the
  private sector? Can the necessary measurement of performance and costs in the private and public sector be
  created?
- Can government further extend coverage of health services to the poor by encouraging and perhaps formalizing
  pro-poor measures being claimed by the private sector?
  Can it effectively monitor health gains by the poor?
- How can government take advantage of opportunities to
  work with private providers? Are there opportunities for
  the public sector to network with alternate private
  providers, even though there are legal constraints on
  untrained medical practice?
- Can governments intervene in areas that would make the
  biggest difference in motivating health workers, notably
  training opportunities?

the role of public infrastructure, and other business constraints are
also examined, including an assessment of transaction costs related
to issues of labor, revenue collection, and regulation. Incentives
and other motivating factors, although not strictly matters of contestability, play a critical role in shaping the behavior of the private
sector, and that role is also explored here. We treat motivation
along with contestability largely because it is important in determining whether an individual will choose to work in the private
sector and how that individual will behave, and because motivation

is not considered a measurable indicator of quality or output of health service.

Some of the most important issues of measurability in the private sector concern performance and pricing. Quality is an important performance factor in health care, so we look at dimensions of quality of care related to staffing, clinical practices, and management of quality as well as patients' perceptions of quality. We also examine the measurability of services provided, outputs, and equity questions, particularly how the poor are treated in private practice.

The studies shed light on the area of private sector interactions with the public sector. They show the degree to which the private sector is already working with the public sector and reveal where greater partnership may be possible. Participation in national programs, opportunities to improve the quality of care or coverage of services, and other areas for collaboration are explored.

Our findings give a better understanding of how the private sector works and provide a basis for governments to make decisions to make-buy-regulate-inform, as described in the preceding chapter, and to provide better oversight of the health sector generally. Such information can reveal areas in which the private sector might benefit from further support as well as areas in which it can or should be left alone. It also generates options for government to overcome private market failures, to form strategic partnerships with the private sector, and to adapt ideas and ways of doing things from the private sector to the public sector.

Context: The Private Health Sector in India

Levels of private financing of health in India are among the highest in the world, meaning that much of health care is already exposed to market conditions. The analysis of health financing in chapters 8 and 9 shows that reliance on individual private payment for health is not only inefficient and less accountable than other methods of financing; it also drastically increases vulnerability to poverty.

Health care in India is also largely provided through the private sector and is highly diverse in methods and quality. The Indian systems of medicine, consisting of the ancient methods of ayurveda, unani, siddha, amchi, naturopathy, and yoga, as well as homeopathy, have always been dominated by private practitioners and private financing, at least in ambulatory care. Doctors trained in Indian systems, about one-fourth of formally trained doctors in India, continue to provide a significant part of the private ambulatory care market.

At the time of independence, most allopathic (Western) medicine was provided through government facilities. Private allopathic medicine was limited to a few missionary hospitals and private industries and thus accounted for only a small part of India's formal health system. Now, however, more than 80 percent of qualified allopathic doctors are based in the private sector.

The picture is complicated by the fact that many public sector doctors also practice privately after hours, either in their own clinics or as consultants in private hospitals. The legality of private practice for public sector doctors differs from state to state, and the frequency of this practice is unknown. In the consultations associated with these studies, most participants familiar with the health sector believed that the majority of public doctors also practiced privately, a belief supported by the few small-area studies that have looked at the question (Chawla 2000).

Most health statistics are limited to the formal sector (the realm of trained practitioners). A reliable estimate of the number of untrained providers does not exist because such practitioners are not registered—the Supreme Court has held their work to be illegal and has labeled them "quacks." Nonetheless, the largest number of health providers in India, estimated at well over 1.25 million, are untrained and are believed to usually practice allopathic medicine or a mix of systems. Unlike the formally trained allopathic doctors, who concentrate in urban areas and larger towns, most untrained providers are found in rural areas, where they are the first source of ambulatory care for the rural poor (Rohde and Viswanathan 1995).

The distribution of private and public services also varies by location and type of service, an indication that the markets are already quite segmented. The private sector offers a relatively small share of preventive services (less than 10 percent of immunizations delivered and 40 percent of prenatal care) but takes a much larger portion of curative services, particularly dominating the provision of ambulatory care (figure 6.1). Results from the 52nd Round of the National Sample Survey reveal that the private sector is generally much more pro-rich in its distribution than the public sector (Background Paper 18). (Chapter 7 provides further analysis of the distribution of different types of health services in different states and across services and poverty groups.) The poor depend largely on the public sector for services, except for ambulatory care, for which all groups overwhelmingly depend on the private sector. Thus a larger private sector is associated with a more pro-poor distribution of public health services.

This chapter addresses the question of how the different segments of the private health sector actually work.

Methods

The illegality of some types of private practice and the general neglect of the private sector by researchers and policymakers have left a gap in the theoretical framework, research tools, and data on the functioning of the private health market. Because no comprehensive registry or sampling frame of private providers exists, and because admission statistics and patient records are rarely available for examination, less desirable methods had to be used for sampling and examining performance in the private sector. The selection of providers, for example, was based on a stratification of districts and random selection of hospitals, which were then used as locators to randomly select qualified private allopathic practitioners—those having an M.D. (Doctor of Medicine) or MBBS (Bachelor of Medicine and Bachelor of Surgery) degree—and the two types of private practitioners that we term "alternative":[1]

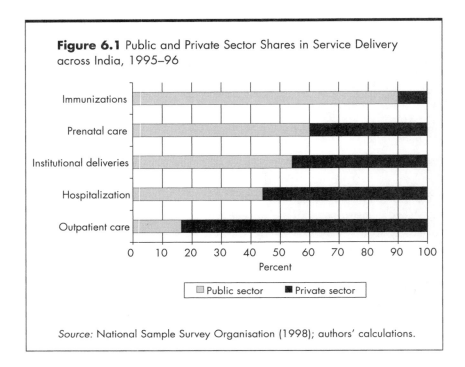

Figure 6.1 Public and Private Sector Shares in Service Delivery across India, 1995–96

Source: National Sample Survey Organisation (1998); authors' calculations.

- Practitioners of Indian systems of medicine (those practicing non-allopathic systems of medicine, most of whom have formal qualifications in a nonallopathic system).

- Untrained allopathic practitioners (those who usually practice allopathic medicine but have no formal training or qualifications in the system of medicine they are practicing).

One consequence of these methods is that the sample selected is more representative of markets having high concentrations of inpatient facilities, which tend to serve urban areas and nearby rural populations. Second, the likelihood of selection is increased for those providers who do more business. This means that the sample tends to represent more successful private providers and to underrepresent providers who work part-time or who are not competing well. The studies may therefore be underestimating some of the problems of

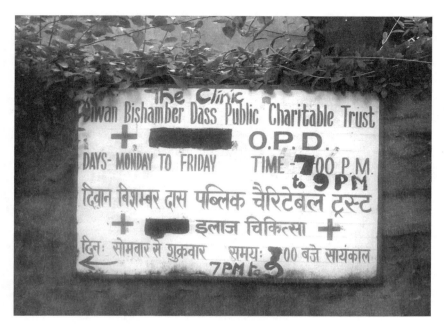

A private clinic (PHOTOGRAPH BY GEETANJALI CHOPRA/THE WORLD BANK)

contestability and are likely to be examining providers who have better quality and measurability. One indicator of the latter point is that among the alternative private providers selected, the proportion of untrained practitioners was lower than in previous studies conducted in rural Uttar Pradesh. In the sample used by Rohde and Viswanathan (1995), just over half the providers had no training, whereas only one-third had no training in the present Uttar Pradesh sample.

Ambulatory Care

The study sampled 71 clinics of qualified allopathic providers in Andhra Pradesh and 86 clinics in Uttar Pradesh. It also sampled 156 alternative private practitioners in Andhra Pradesh and 84 in Uttar Pradesh. Of the alternative practitioners in Andhra Pradesh, 44 percent claimed to practice allopathic medicine, compared with 30 percent in the Uttar Pradesh sample. Homeopathy was the most common system of medicine used in Uttar Pradesh (57 percent of all sampled alternative practitioners) and the second most common system after allopathy in Andhra Pradesh (35 percent). Ayurveda was the third most frequent system of medicine used in both states. Practicing more than one system of medicine is relatively common (34 percent in Andhra Pradesh, 19 percent in Uttar Pradesh), usually a combination of allopathy and ayurveda. An additional fifth of those claiming to practice nonallopathic medicines actually provide allopathic therapies to their patients (see p. 164).

Contestability

Among the qualified allopathic practitioners in both states, nearly all were established as proprietary, for-profit clinics, averaging 13 years of practice. The alternative private practitioners also had well-established practices, averaging 14 years duration in Andhra Pradesh and 13 years in Uttar Pradesh. About 80 percent of alternative private practitioners in both states worked full time as medical practitioners, almost always alone. Likewise, the qualified allopaths practiced ambulatory care in solo clinics. In both states, the main motivation stated by alternative private practitioners for entering practice was to provide a service for those in need. In Andhra Pradesh and among nonallopathic practitioners in Uttar Pradesh, carrying out a family tradition was the next most common reason, whereas the untrained practitioners in Uttar Pradesh cited a good income as the second most common reason (appendix table 6A.1).

The capital needed to operate a clinic is often minimal—only a room and a limited amount of equipment and drugs are needed. Low-cost items such as thermometers, stethoscopes, and blood pressure equipment were nearly always present in such clinics.

Patient consultations are the main source of income for nearly 90 percent of all alternative private practitioners. This pattern suggests that the traditional practice of charging little or nothing for a consultation but building a margin into medicines may have changed over the past decade (Rohde and Viswanathan 1995). In any case, the incomes of most alternative private practitioners we sampled are now comfortably middle class. Among the alternative providers, the nonallopathic practitioners earned more than Rs 8,000 per month on average, compared with less than Rs 5,000 per month on average for the untrained allopathic practitioners.

Only a few alternative private practitioners received money for referring patients to a facility (table 6.1). Pharmaceutical representatives have extensively penetrated the alternative private practitioner market in Andhra Pradesh, where nearly all alternative private practitioners benefited from free samples of drugs. More than one-third of the untrained practitioners received compensation from drug companies that was tied to their patients' use of pharmaceutical products, compared with about one-tenth of the nonallopathic practitioners. In Uttar Pradesh, where the association of pharmaceutical companies with alternative private practitioners is not as great, the practice of kickbacks for use of a pharmaceutical product was more common and indicated a more aggressive marketing strategy by the pharmaceutical companies.

The data presented here suggest that barriers to entry are quite low in the ambulatory care market. Given the absence of any licensing or accreditation, and without enforcement of regulations concerning

Table 6.1 Alternative Private Practitioners Receiving Informal Payments, Andhra Pradesh and Uttar Pradesh

(percent)

	ANDHRA PRADESH		UTTAR PRADESH	
TYPE OF PAYMENT	UNTRAINED ALLOPATHIC PRACTITIONERS	NONALLOPATHIC PRACTITIONERS	UNTRAINED ALLOPATHIC PRACTITIONERS	NONALLOPATHIC PRACTITIONERS
Cash for patient referrals	7	8	8	14
Free drug samples	86	80	60	56
Rewards for patients' use of products[a]	35	13	52	27

a. For Andhra Pradesh, statistically significant at $p < 0.01$; for Uttar Pradesh, at $p < 0.05$.
Source: Background Papers 20 and 21; authors' calculations.

educational standards or physical standards, nearly anyone can set up shop as a doctor. The capital requirements for ambulatory clinics are also minimal, and so is the need for access to credit or infrastructure. As a result, the ambulatory care market is often quite competitive. Although their stated motivations are frequently altruistic, practitioners are subject to influence by pharmaceutical companies.

Although few steps have been taken to alter the contestability of the ambulatory care market, it could be done by encouraging qualified practitioners to serve markets in which greater needs exist (for example, through special subsidies) or by restricting the entry of low-quality providers through rigorous licensing or accreditation. Nonetheless, the main constraints to influencing the ambulatory care market lie in the area of measurability.

Measurability

Here we present previously unavailable measurements of the work of outpatient care providers. We first look at information on the workload of private providers, including the number of patients and type of clinical conditions seen. We then examine the prices charged for outpatient consultations in different settings. We conclude by discussing what can be learned from measurements of quality of care and of the relationship of ambulatory care practice to the poor.

Service data. Although data are now available on the rates of outpatient consultations in the private sector (see chapter 7), little is known about the workload of private practices, or about the type of patients seen by the private health provider. Data gathered by the present studies show that qualified allopathic practitioners in Andhra Pradesh saw an average of 14 patients per day, compared with 18 patients per day in Uttar Pradesh. These rates are similar to those for alternative private practitioners in the two states: 18 patients per day in Andhra Pradesh and 14 patients per day in Uttar Pradesh, with no statistically significant difference between the untrained allopathic doctors and the nonallopathic doctors. Although both allopathic and nonallopathic practitioners treat a high proportion of common ailments such as fever, cough, diarrhea, pain, skin conditions, and sexual problems, some important differences exist. In both states, the nonallopathic practitioners saw more chronic cases, such as diabetes, and in Uttar Pradesh, they had a larger share of the market for skin disease, hypertension, and sexual problems. The untrained practitioners also had a bigger portion of the market for cases of fever, diarrhea, and deliveries in Andhra Pradesh (appendix table 6A.2).

Pricing. Untrained allopathic practitioners charged far less than any other type of practitioner in either state (appendix table 6A.3). In Andhra Pradesh, the nonallopathic practitioners charged about the same per consultation as allopathic generalists but less than specialists. In Uttar Pradesh, the allopathic generalists charged about three times as much as the nonallopathic doctors in an outpatient setting. Among qualified allopathic practitioners, the generalists charged less than the specialists. We also compared the prices of consultation with the fees charged for outpatient visits to small and large hospitals. In both states, the specialist doctors charged considerably more than anyone else and were more expensive at larger facilities. However, in Andhra Pradesh, generalist doctors charged about the same amount per consultation at small and big hospitals, which was about one-third higher than the rates charged by the same category of provider at outpatient clinics. Similarly, generalist doctors did not attract high fees at the big hospitals in Uttar Pradesh, although the large hospitals tended to rely on the more expensive specialist doctors.

These data suggest that market forces have already differentiated the types of providers in the two states. The untrained allopathic practitioners are placing their fees at a much more affordable level for the poor, whereas other providers can attract higher fees and incomes. The fact that nonallopathic doctors charge the same fees as generalist allopathic doctors in Andhra Pradesh, but less in Uttar Pradesh, suggests that these markets have developed quite differently, either because of differences in the public's expectations or because of differences in the type, quality, or availability of services.

Similarly, the markets in both states are allowing for considerably higher fees for specialists and hospital-based providers.

Quality of care. Without good medical records or the ability to observe patients being cared for in an ambulatory setting, measurements of the quality of care in private outpatient clinics are difficult. One way to examine quality is to look at what types of medicines are used. Some 10–20 percent of the homeopaths and ayurvedic doctors used allopathic medicine despite their being unqualified to do so (appendix table 6A.4). Among the untrained allopathic doctors in both states, the majority used drugs, such as injectable antibiotics and steroids, that should require a prescription. Contraceptives and condoms were relatively uncommon.

We were able to study 1,800 randomly selected prescriptions given by qualified allopathic doctors in Uttar Pradesh and two other states (Tamil Nadu and Karnataka). The average prescription contained more than 3.6 different formulations, compared with 3.0 in the public sector. These results are a crude indicator of overuse of drugs in both private and public sectors. No exact standards exist for the limitation of polypharmacy (the concurrent use of several drugs), especially in the absence of data on the patient's clinical conditions; nonetheless, in most cases no more than two drugs are needed to treat a condition. More drugs are usually unnecessary, difficult to administer, and likely to lead to unwanted drug interactions. Prescribing multiple drugs does, however, raise the income of the pharmacist; it also raises the doctor's income if the doctor has a stake in profits from the drugs prescribed.

The conclusion of irrational drug use in both the public and private sectors is supported by the further analysis of prescriptions given for diarrhea. Every one of the prescriptions for diarrhea in each state included antibiotics or antimotility drugs, although the use of such drugs in the common acute diarrhea seen in outpatient settings is not usually indicated (WHO 1995). The data support the view that rational use of drugs is an important area for improving the quality of care by both public and private providers.

Other indicators showed that patient safety is a problem among some alternative private providers. No sterilizer was found in a considerable proportion of clinics that had an operating theatre (20 percent in Andhra Pradesh, 29 percent in Uttar Pradesh) nor in an even larger proportion of clinics that offered antibiotic injections (35 percent in Andhra Pradesh, 70 percent in Uttar Pradesh). Not surprisingly, practitioners in these clinics were not trained to conduct surgery or give injectable antibiotics. If nothing else, these conditions place patients at risk for diseases such as hepatitis B and HIV. Given such practices, treatment guidelines, provider education, and education of the public may be useful in improving the safety of the public.

The appropriate use of diagnostic services such as radiology, microbiology, or hematology is another important consideration in the quality of ambulatory care that is difficult to measure in India. In our studies, a large difference in the use of diagnostic centers was found among the different types of providers in Andhra Pradesh. Nearly all (91 percent) of the untrained doctors referred patients to diagnostic centers, whereas just over half (56 percent) of the nonallopathic doctors referred patients to diagnostic centers. In Uttar Pradesh, about three-fourths of both types of alternative private practitioners referred patients to diagnostic centers. More detailed studies are needed to examine whether the particular use of diagnostic centers is appropriate or whether it merely generates more revenue for physicians. However, a systematic lack of referral to diagnostic centers by some practitioners suggests that nonreferring providers do not have a strong basis for making a diagnosis or monitoring progress among their patients, since most clinics do not have a wide range of diagnostic equipment to do the tests themselves.

The poor and the private market. The evidence shows that across India the poor overwhelmingly rely on the private sector for ambulatory curative care (chapter 7). Virtually all providers stated that they offered some concessions to the poor (appendix table 6A.5). For the alternative private practitioners, giving such concessions is consistent with the reasons they gave for entering medical practice. Nearly one-third (29 percent) of all patients seen by alternative private practitioners in Andhra Pradesh received some kind of concession because of poverty; the rate was lower in Uttar Pradesh (17 percent).

In both states, free care was the most common type of concession, followed by the provision of free samples in Andhra Pradesh and discounted prices in Uttar Pradesh. Traditional mechanisms for making concessions to the poor, such as deferred payment or payment in kind, were quite rare, as was the offer of less expensive care. The only statistically significant difference between types of practitioners in Andhra Pradesh was that nonallopaths were more likely to offer free samples of medicines than the untrained allopathic practitioners, whereas in Uttar Pradesh, the nonallopaths were more likely to offer free care. However, records on concessions given to the poor were not actually maintained by these providers.

As for the qualified allopaths, nearly all offered concessions to poor patients. However, the pattern of their concessions is different between the two states and in contrast to the pattern of alternative private practitioners' concessions. Among qualified allopaths in Uttar Pradesh, free samples of medicine and free care are much more commonly used than any other method; discount prices and deferred payment were other common methods in Andhra Pradesh.

These data show that the private market is sensitive to the economic condition of the poor and may help explain why the poor rely on the private sector for ambulatory care. Other studies have suggested that the convenient clinic hours, helpful attitudes of providers, availability of medicines, and knowledge that the provider is a longstanding member of the community are often reasons why the private sector is preferred over the public sector (Rohde and Viswanathan 1995). Within a given market area, these factors and the ability to give concessions to the poor may well give a provider an edge over competitors.

Whether giving concessions to the poor is considered a profit-maximizing behavior or a commitment to the community is a difficult question to test or monitor, especially because treatment for the poor is not well measured. The alternative private practitioners studied did not keep records on the type of concessions given to the poor. As for the qualified allopathic clinics, less than 10 percent of them in Andhra Pradesh had records on assistance given to the poor, while none of them in Uttar Pradesh had such records.

Interaction with the Public Sector

Private sector participation in various national health programs in the two states is quite variable. Broadly viewed, however, the level of reported participation in national programs is much lower than the levels of expressed desire to participate; participation usually occurs through the Pulse Polio campaigns or by referring patients for family planning (table 6.2). Given the Supreme Court ruling requiring state governments to crack down on medical quackery, careful thought is needed when exploring the partnerships that may be possible with untrained medical practitioners. Nonetheless, among the alternative private practitioners, the disparity between their expressed desire to participate and their actual participation in national programs suggests a number of potentially useful opportunities for partnerships (see box 6.2).

In Andhra Pradesh, the alternative private practitioners also reported having a high opinion of public health and family planning programs, particularly in contrast to their views of government inpatient and outpatient services (appendix table 6A.6). However, alternative private practitioners in Uttar Pradesh have a much poorer opinion of government programs. This suggests that in Andhra Pradesh there is a greater opportunity to increase the coverage of national programs by further involving alternative providers. In Uttar Pradesh, there may be a larger credibility gap with the alternative private practitioners.

More than one-half of the alternative private practitioners in Andhra Pradesh belong to professional associations (and about 40 percent in Uttar Pradesh); the majority of members say they find the groups to be useful. They say that training and the setting of guidelines by the associations would be particularly welcome (figure 6.2)—both would provide practical ways to induce alternative pri-

Box 6.2 Working with Untrained Private Providers: The Janani Experience

Most health care to the rural poor is provided through alternative private practitioners (APPs), a group that consists of non-allopathic practitioners and untrained allopathic providers. In the states of Bihar and Jarkhand, the number of APPs is estimated at between 200,000 and 250,000. Janani, a nonprofit social marketing and reproductive health services organization, decided that the only way to reach the rural poor with reproductive health services was through the huge army of APPs. To do so, Janani launched a novel project to franchise reproductive health services in Bihar through a network of APPs.

The rural providers, however, were not interested in selling condoms and oral contraceptives, the only two methods they are legally allowed to sell, as the returns were too low. Janani estimated that in a village of 2,000, the monthly income from providing all the contraceptive needs would be about Rs 2, not enough to buy a cup of tea.

Janani's strategy is to bundle services to make the participation of rural providers into a viable network. Janani's program attempts to offer the entire range of reproductive health services, and uses a franchisee network of urban clinics run by qualified doctors for referral. APPs are trained to identify reproductive-tract infections, do pregnancy tests, and offer referral to qualified urban-based allopaths who are also part of the network. One qualified doctor provides back-up for 20 APPs. Advertising of the plan is built around the "Butterfly" logo that is displayed at the franchisee's place.

Clients pay a fixed fee for all services. For every client referred to the urban doctors, who are franchised by Janani under a "Rising Sun" logo, the rural providers earn an attractive commission. In exchange for participating in the Janani "Butterfly" network and deriving benefits from the aggressive marketing and promotional campaign, the rural providers have to sell condoms and oral contraceptives at all times.

To have a significant effect on reproductive health (and be financially rewarding to the rural providers) the program has to be accommodating to women clients. Toward that end the Janani network requires that each rural provider invited to join the Janani network be, or include, a woman (the partnerships are typically among family members). The women of the community gain the comfort of being able to deal with another woman regarding reproductive health; and the provider partnership gains more business and more income by being able to offer that accommodation.

Through its aggressive advertising and promotions, the Janani program creates the impression that the "Butterfly" network of rural providers is prestigious and economically rewarding to its members. All rural providers pay a yearly fee of Rs 500. But to encourage adherence to the strictly enforced norms of the network, the rural providers can earn discounts on the fee (of up to 50 percent) according to how closely they operate their clinics to Janani's prescribed standards.

The success of the program hinges on an effective management structure, and the current challenge of the Janani program is not establishing its networks but sustaining them. Janani's plan is to keep the organization thin and streamlined. Its role is increasingly becoming one of oversight rather than implementation. Almost all the fieldwork is outsourced, and competition among rival entrepreneurs is used as the way to monitor and implement. With regard to monitoring, most of the quantifiable indicators are tied to money to create strong pressures within the management system.

The program has had much success since its beginning in 1996. From the outset, Janani intended to include two APPs per panchayat, or about 24,000 providers. Janani has already recruited 16,000 APPs and is expected to cover all the panchayats by the end of 2001. During 2000, the network provided contraception for 1 million couple years.

Table 6.2 Participation in National Health Programs by Private Practitioners, Andhra Pradesh and Uttar Pradesh

(percent)

PARTICIPATION	ANDHRA PRADESH			UTTAR PRADESH		
	UNTRAINED ALLOPATH	NONALLOPATH	QUALIFIED ALLOPATH	UNTRAINED ALLOPATH	NONALLOPATH	QUALIFIED ALLOPATH
Desires to participate in national programs	81	64	31	48	39	61
Does participate in particular national programs						
Family planning program	42	10	27	24	27	51
Polio eradication program	38	24	31	36	44	69
Malaria control program	25	13	21	8	9	16
Blindness control program	21	8	17	8	2	5
HIV/AIDS control program	19	13	21	8	10	48
Tuberculosis control program	18	13	17	9	0	41
Leprosy control program	12	10	10	8	7	1

Source: Background Papers 20 and 21; authors' calculations.

vate practitioners to participate in national programs, to improve the quality of the care they give, to better network with the public sector, and to refer patients as needed.

Overall, the present studies point out that despite substantial variation among market locations, the public sector has many opportunities to work in partnership with private ambulatory care providers. The kinds of partnership activities that are welcome cost little money, but they take time and effort. The benefits that may result include improved quality of care, greater coverage for health interventions of national priority, and better communications and sharing of information among providers (see appendix D for a list of efforts to address the role of private providers in national tuberculosis control progams).

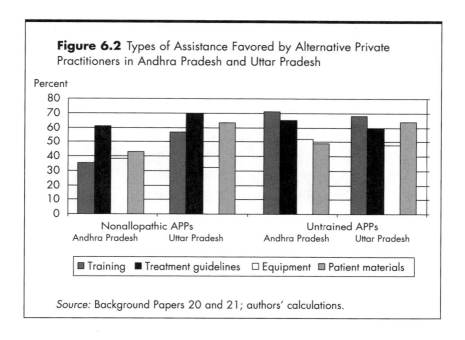

Figure 6.2 Types of Assistance Favored by Alternative Private Practitioners in Andhra Pradesh and Uttar Pradesh

Source: Background Papers 20 and 21; authors' calculations.

Inpatient Care

The studies examined two types of private inpatient facilities, using public sector hospitals for comparison where possible:

- Small hospitals (facilities having fewer than 50 beds), commonly called nursing homes.

- Large hospitals (those having at least 100 beds).

The sample covered 69 small hospitals and 10 large hospitals in Andhra Pradesh, and 64 small hospitals and 12 large hospitals in Uttar Pradesh. The number of private sector health personnel interviewed was 331 in Andhra Pradesh and 421 in Uttar Pradesh. The number of private patients interviewed was 1,175 in Andhra Pradesh and 1,620 in Uttar Pradesh.[2]

Contestability

Issues of contestability generally loom larger for the inpatient market than for ambulatory care: the investment and maintenance costs are much greater, hospitals have a higher public profile, and inpatient operations are more complex. In this section, therefore, we go into more detail in examining how hospitals have been established and expanded over time. We take a more comprehensive look at the issues of costs of credit, labor problems, constraints of public infrastructure, and the regulatory environment. Finally, we examine the questions of motivation of workers in more detail than we did in the previous section.

In both Andhra Pradesh and Uttar Pradesh, most private hospitals were established in the 1980s. Nearly all the small hospitals sampled in both states are incorporated as proprietary companies, largely to provide their owners with a facility in which to practice medicine. In both states, half of the large hospitals were nonprofit hospitals incorporated as a trust or society.

Financial factors. To get established, most hospitals in both states required a start-up loan, usually from a commercial bank or other private source. Access to finance was relatively easy for most hospitals (appendix table 6A.7). The most significant obstacles to credit cited by hospital owners and managers were the amount of paperwork required for loans and high interest rates.

The private hospitals sampled, particularly in Uttar Pradesh, tend to continue to invest in their business and expand (appendix table 6A.8). Virtually all the private hospitals have grown in numbers of beds since they were established, although the floor-space per bed is considerably smaller than that found in the public sector. Another indication of growth is that, at the time of the sampling, the majority of private hospitals in Uttar Pradesh had invested in buildings during the past year, and about four-fifths had invested in equipment. More than half expected to make capital investments in the next year as well. As was the case with initial financing, government played a negligible role in providing financing for investment in private hospitals in both states, with private sources predominating.

Regarding cash flow, we found that the vast majority of private hospitals sampled are meeting their operating costs from their revenues (appendix table 6A.9), the largest share of which almost always comes from patient fees. More than three-fourths of facilities report rising revenues. These results are in part related to the study design, which biased selection toward facilities with more patients and away from failing facilities. Nonetheless, most small hospitals complained of significant competition from other hospitals, which may be desirable from a public policy perspective. In Andhra Pradesh, nonpayment was a frequent problem for nearly two-thirds of small hospitals and for one-third of large hospitals, whereas hospitals in Uttar Pradesh were more likely to complain of having too few paying patients. The studies have also demonstrated that private hospitals are able to reduce costs by using significantly smaller buildings than are used in the public sector and by keeping down the number of paramedical and support staff, factors that may also reduce the quality of care.

Business environment. On the question of labor constraints, the studies found that low productivity, an absence of skilled workers, and the high cost of skilled employees are the most significant problems with labor in private hospitals (appendix table 6A.10). Surprisingly, problems between management and unions, regulations on working conditions, and restrictions on laying off workers—all issues that often constrain management action in the public sector—are relatively minor concerns in the private sector.

Private hospital owners in both states view problems with the public infrastructure, especially drainage, telecommunications, and electricity, as more important than labor issues (appendix table 6A.11). As would be expected given their different levels of development, infrastructure problems are larger in Uttar Pradesh than in Andhra Pradesh.

General regulatory issues are a much more significant problem for private hospitals in Uttar Pradesh than in Andhra Pradesh (appendix table 6A.12). In both states, the largest constraint is reported to be high taxes. In Uttar Pradesh, problems with the judicial system are cited as the next most common regulatory constraint, followed by tax administration, whereas in Andhra Pradesh, obtaining government clearances is ranked second. The relatively low level of difficulty with quality standards and price controls reflects the absence of intervention in these areas by government or professional bodies.

These findings show that contestability issues are important for the private hospital sector in the two states. The data suggest that most private hospitals are succeeding financially and are expanding. Among the private hospitals studied for this report, credit has not been a major constraint. In any case, few private hospitals needed financial help from the government. Instead, as demonstrated by their continued investment in equipment, private hospitals tended to rely on banks and their own private resources to expand their size or services. Unless one takes the view that steps are needed to encourage more private hospitals to enter the market, expanded access to credit is unlikely to improve contestability in the private hospital sector. On the other hand, the most important business constraints appear to be related to public infrastructure and the regulatory environment, particularly in Uttar Pradesh. Improvements in these areas have greater potential for improving contestability in the private hospital sector.

Motivations of Providers

Before turning to questions of measurability, we will examine some of the important motivators of participants in the public and private sectors. People who practice in the public health sector are often assumed to be motivated by factors other than those motivating private health practitioners. In particular, money is said to motivate those in the private sector, and security those in the public sector.[3] Rather than dwell on these stereotypes, we examined the extent to which the motivating factors reported by health providers were actually present in their work. Seventeen types of motivating factors were studied; they were grouped into the categories of work environment, professional fulfillment, work relationships, and personal benefits.

The study results reveal relatively few differences between public and private sector health workers in the motivations they say are important (appendix table 6A.13). In Andhra Pradesh, having good working relationships with colleagues, good physical working conditions, and challenging work that offers a sense of accomplishment are the most important motivating factors for public and private sector providers. In Uttar Pradesh, good working relationships with colleagues is most important for public and private sector providers, although private sector providers consider good physical working conditions and training opportunities as the next most important factors, whereas public sector workers rank availability of tools for work and career advancement as next most important. Notably, having a good income or job security is not rated highly by either public sector or private sector workers.

Nonetheless, some important differences exist in the factors that motivate public and private sector health workers. Using multivariate regression analysis to examine the differences between public and private sector health workers, and adjusting for the effects of profession, type of health facility, age, and sex, four significant differences were found among the motivating factors in the Andhra Pradesh sample. Compared with private sector health workers, public sector health workers attach significantly higher importance to employment benefits, opportunities to advance to a better job, and having a superior who recognizes their work. Private sector workers rate the importance of being respected and trusted by clients significantly higher than do public sector workers. No significant difference emerged between the two groups in the importance of income or job security, which were rated lower than other common factors.

An examination of the degree to which health workers believe that motivating factors are actually present in their work revealed greater differences than were found in their stated ideals (appendix table 6A.14). The first observation is that ways to improve working conditions can be discovered from the fact that the rating for the actual presence of each motivating factor is much lower than its desired presence. There are also many more differences between the public and private sectors. Using the same types of multivariate models, we found that the public and private sectors differ significantly on eight parameters (appendix table 6A.15). In Andhra Pradesh, private sector workers rate their physical working conditions as significantly better than those in the public sector and report less political interference. Curiously, public and private sector workers report a similar level of need to pay bribes to accomplish things. Private sector workers also report having more tools and materials to do their work, feel they have greater respect from their clients, and are more likely to be based in a desirable location and have a good income. Public sector workers have higher ratings for having a superior recognize their work and having good employment benefits.

The results also pointed out some relevant gender differences in motivating factors. Women rate having sufficient time for personal or family life significantly higher than men do, whereas men rate having challenging work that offers a sense of accomplishment and being respected by clients significantly higher than women do. With regard to actual working conditions, the differences between men and women are even greater. Men rate their working conditions better than women do on five parameters, while women did not rate any conditions more highly than men did. Men reported having better training opportunities, more tools to do their job, more respect from clients, more independence from interference by superiors, and better incomes.

We also examined the level of unmet needs by looking at the disparity between reports of ideal job characteristics and the degree to which those characteristics were reported to be present in the current job. This analysis may be used to design interventions to influence health worker behavior. The first observation is that the disparity between ideal and actual job characteristics among private sector workers is significantly smaller than among public sector workers. High income and job security rate relatively low as unmet needs, possibly because they are found to be satisfactorily present among 43 percent of private employees and 48 percent of public employees. Among the top five motivating factors in both the public and private sectors, only training opportunities are a top source of disparity in both Andhra Pradesh and Uttar Pradesh. Otherwise, the largest disparity is among factors that are rated as less important. However, what is notable in the public sector in Uttar Pradesh is that the largest disparity involves the problems of corrupt practices and political interference in decisionmaking.

These findings suggest that those who work in the public and private sectors have similar ideals but that large differences exist in how well employment in the public and private sectors satisfies those ideals. Reassuringly, the results also point out that income is not among the most important factors in meeting worker expectations, indicating that other interventions may have a greater effect on satisfaction than raising personal incomes. Training opportunities are among the most straightforward and highly sought-after interventions that would satisfy health workers in both sectors.

Measurability

As they do for the ambulatory care market, questions of measurability loom larger than those of contestability. Here, we look at some of the main issues of measurability related to services, prices, quality, and dealings with the poor.

Service data. In Andhra Pradesh, small private hospitals tended to provide a more limited range of clinical services than did small public hospitals, whereas large private hospitals were more comprehensive than large public hospitals. For example, family planning services were provided at 76 percent of small private hospitals and 91 percent of large private hospitals; the same services were provided at all small public hospitals but at just 44 percent of large public hospitals. Twenty-four-hour emergency services were offered at 60 percent of small private hospitals and 82 percent of large private hospitals; the same services were offered at 94 percent of small public hospitals and 67 percent of large public hospitals. Diagnostic services such as biochemistry, microbiology, ultrasound, and computerized tomography scanning are all more commonly available at private hospitals. Patterns in the range of services offered at private facilities in Uttar Pradesh were similar to those found in Andhra Pradesh.

Staffing patterns also affect the type and quality of services provided, and they vary between the two states (appendix table 6A.16). In Andhra Pradesh, where private practice by government doctors is legal, the number of part-time government doctors (almost all specialists) reported to be working in large hospitals is large. In Uttar Pradesh, where private practice by government doctors is not permitted, relatively few are reported to practice in private hospitals. General medical duty officers nearly always work full time at hospitals and are rarely government doctors.

The number of beds covered by doctors and nurses varies considerably between the states and by size of hospital (figure 6.3). Hospitals in Andhra Pradesh have a much higher number of beds per doctor and per nurse than do those in Uttar Pradesh. The number of nurses is exceptionally low in both states, raising serious questions about the ability to provide quality nursing care. Accounting for three shifts of nurses in a day would mean that one qualified nurse would be expected to care for patients in more than 80 beds at one time in large hospitals in Andhra Pradesh, a ratio that allows for less than 6 minutes of care per patient per day.

Regarding surgery, most patients are in a poor position to assess whether surgery is needed or to know who provides the best surgery. Surgery can also be a major source of revenue for a hospital. High rates of surgery may indicate greater specialization by a hospital, but they can also suggest supplier-induced demand for unnecessary services. Without being able to assess the type of cases seen, their severity, and their clinical outcomes, judgments about the appropriateness of care or its quality cannot easily be made.

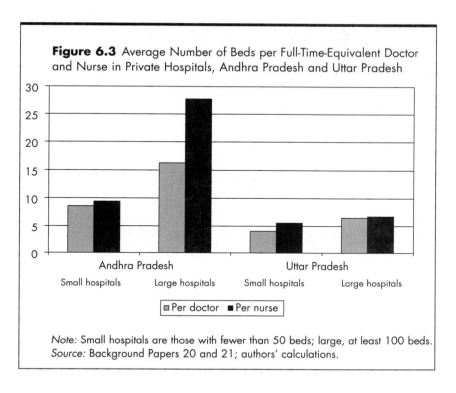

Figure 6.3 Average Number of Beds per Full-Time-Equivalent Doctor and Nurse in Private Hospitals, Andhra Pradesh and Uttar Pradesh

Note: Small hospitals are those with fewer than 50 beds; large, at least 100 beds.
Source: Background Papers 20 and 21; authors' calculations.

Cesarean sections (births delivered surgically) constitute one of the few areas in which some judgment can be made on the appropriateness of surgery in the absence of full clinical information. Although no international standard exists, hospitals with cesarean section rates above 15–20 percent are likely to be overusing the procedure. Yet in the present studies, nearly one-third of all hospital deliveries were cesarean (table 6.3). Such a rate is especially likely to represent overuse because the hospitals examined are not tertiary care institutions, to which women with high-risk pregnancies would have been referred and where higher rates of cesarean section would therefore be expected.[4]

Other common measures of hospital performance include bed-occupancy rate and average length of stay. Confident interpretations of such data would require further information on the mix of cases seen or on the outcomes of care. Nonetheless, low bed-occupancy rates

Table 6.3 Performance Indicators of Private Hospitals, Andhra Pradesh and Uttar Pradesh, 2000

INDICATOR	ANDHRA PRADESH		UTTAR PRADESH	
	SMALL HOSPITALS	LARGE HOSPITALS	SMALL HOSPITALS	LARGE HOSPITALS
Bed occupancy rate (percent)	40	64	41	42
Average length of stay (days)	6.2	5.5	3.9	5.5
Cesarean section rate (percent)	29.7	29.3	30.1	36.4
Major surgeries per specialist doctor (annual)	36.7	107.4	55.1	92.9

Note: Small hospitals are those with fewer than 50 beds; large, at least 100 beds.
Source: Background Papers 20 and 21; authors' calculations.

show that the private hospitals are operating far below their capacity and that, in general, they are not keeping beds full through long stays. Bed-occupancy rates are slightly higher in small private hospitals than in public hospitals in the same areas, and stays are marginally shorter (STEM 2000). Among large hospitals in Andhra Pradesh, the public sector has a higher bed occupancy than the private sector; among large hospitals in Uttar Pradesh, the opposite is the case.

Quality. Available information about the appropriateness of staffing levels and the physical size of facilities provides some indication of limitations in the quality of private hospital services. In addition, the study specifically examined quality assurance processes. Overall, little recording and analysis of health information occur at private health facilities. Few private facilities use clinical protocols, although considerably more claim to maintain medical records, review deaths, and use a patient referral policy (table 6.4). In providing more comprehensive services, the private sector did relatively well. Twenty-four-hour emergency and ambulance services are nearly always provided at private hospitals in Uttar Pradesh and at large hospitals in Andhra Pradesh; they are less likely to be found in small hospitals in Andhra Pradesh.

Table 6.4 Quality Assurance Standards in Hospitals, Andhra Pradesh and Uttar Pradesh
(percent)

| | ANDHRA PRADESH | | | | UTTAR PRADESH | |
| | SMALL HOSPITALS | | LARGE HOSPITALS | | SMALL HOSPITALS | LARGE HOSPITALS |
INDICATOR	PUBLIC	PRIVATE	PUBLIC	PRIVATE	PRIVATE	PRIVATE
Uses clinical protocols	57	23	62	50	31	33
Keeps medical records for more than 3 years	—	—	—	—	66	75
Has procedure to review deaths	—	54	—	100	66	75
Has referral policy	91	78	82	70	84	75
24-hour emergency service	57	67	73	80	91	100
Ambulance service	36	23	91	80	83	100
Cesarean section rate of less than 20 percent	—	27	—	29	25	10

— Nor available.
Note: Small hospitals are those with fewer than 50 beds; large, at least 100 beds.
Source: Background Papers 20 and 21; authors' calculations.

Hospital managers were quite attuned to the need to improve the quality of care (table 6.5). In particular, managers preferred less invasive forms of improvement, such as continuing medical education, hospital quality assurance, doctor and hospital registration, and voluntary accreditation by a nongovernmental organization. Compulsory accreditation through the government was not seen as a good option.

Patient satisfaction is another important dimension of quality assurance. As a routine tool for quality assurance, patient satisfaction surveys are still not commonly used in the private sector, although they are being introduced in the public sector. Some interesting findings on overall satisfaction with services emerged in Andhra Pradesh (table 6.6). Satisfaction was much higher among users of private sector facilities. The private sector seems most able to satisfy the richest quintile of patients. Public facilities failed to satisfy users from the wealthiest 60 percent of the patients.

Table 6.5 Private Hospitals Whose Managers Favor Various Procedures for Improving Hospital Quality, 2000
(percent)

PROCEDURE	ANDHRA PRADESH		UTTAR PRADESH	
	SMALL HOSPITALS	LARGE HOSPITALS	SMALL HOSPITALS	LARGE HOSPITALS
Hospital registration	89	88	75	92
Renewing hospital registration	73	88	55	82
Registering doctors	92	88	88	92
Renewing doctors' registration	77	88	50	73
Voluntary hospital accreditation by NGO	62	83	75	83
Compulsory hospital accreditation by government	44	57	30	58
Hospital quality assurance programs	84	88	89	100
Continuing education for doctors	95	100	97	100

Note: Small hospitals are those with fewer than 50 beds; large, at least 100 beds.
Source: Background Paper 20; authors' calculations.

The poor and the private market. In their dealings with the poor, private inpatient facilities show results similar to those for private providers of ambulatory care. Nearly all private hospitals claim to make concessions for poor patients (table 6.7). However, the pattern of concessions differs between the states and by practitioner. Discount pricing, rather than free care, is the most common type of concession among hospitals. Free samples of medicine are less common in Andhra Pradesh than Uttar Pradesh, and less expensive care is a more likely option in Uttar Pradesh hospitals than it is for any other private provider. These differences in methods for dealing with the poor make standard approaches and measurement of assistance more difficult.

Despite these concessions, the clients served by the private sector are generally not the poor. In both Andhra Pradesh and Uttar Pradesh, the public sector sees significantly higher proportions of poor patients than the private sector, although the private sector also sees more patients (see chapter 7). In Andhra Pradesh, for example,

Table 6.6 Proportion of Patients Satisfied or Very Satisfied with Overall Quality of Care at Public and Private Health Facilities, Andhra Pradesh, by Type of Facility and Wealth of Patient

(percent)

FACILITY OR INCOME QUINTILE	PUBLIC FACILITIES (1)	PRIVATE FACILITIES (2)	PRIVATE-PUBLIC RATIO, (2)/(1)
Clinics and primary health centers	13	30	2.2
Small hospitals	16	23	1.4
Large hospitals	10	29	2.8
Income quintile			
1 (lowest)	20	24	1.2
2	16	14	0.9
3	9	20	2.2
4	13	22	1.8
5 (highest)	8	33	3.9

Note: Small hospitals are those with fewer than 50 beds; large, at least 100 beds.
Source: Background Papers 20 and 21; authors' calculations.

Table 6.7 Private Hospitals Offering Concessions to the Poor, Andhra Pradesh and Uttar Pradesh

(percent)

TYPE OF CONCESSION	ANDHRA PRADESH SMALL HOSPITALS	ANDHRA PRADESH LARGE HOSPITALS	UTTAR PRADESH SMALL HOSPITALS	UTTAR PRADESH LARGE HOSPITALS
Any	99	80	100	100
Free care	74	50	81	75
Free samples of medicine	62	30	81	92
Discount prices	71	60	88	92
Deferred payment	33	20	52	50
Less expensive care	26	20	53	83
Payment in kind	9	10	11	17

Note: Small hospitals are those with fewer than 50 beds; large, at least 100 beds.
Source: Background Papers 20 and 21; authors' calculations.

the proportion of patients seen at small hospitals in the public sector decreases with each rise in wealth quintile, whereas it rises in the private sector. In practice, the private hospitals are catering to a wealthier consumer than the public sector.

The data shown here indicate that the measurement of activities, prices, and performance is particularly weak in the private hospitals studied.

- Most hospitals are quite casual about the setting of fees, allowing doctors to set their own.

- Tariffs are frequently not published, making it more difficult for the consumer to compare prices or to know what to expect.

- Most patients believe that the billing at private facilities is fair.

- No formal system exists for determining exemptions or concessions to the poor; the doctor is nearly always the one who decides whether a patient should be given a concession.

- Few facilities keep records on the concessions they make to the poor.

- The majority of hospitals claim to maintain medical records for at least three years, but the quality of those records is questionable.

- Few private hospitals actually collate records on service outputs, diseases and conditions, or clinical outcomes, suggesting that internal clinical quality assurance mechanisms are largely nonexistent and that vital information is not available to consumers and government planners.

Improving the measurability of the private sector is clearly important if public intervention is to make the health system more accountable, efficient, and pro-poor.

In the next section, we examine interactions between the public and private hospital sectors and explore some opportunities for action.

Interaction with the Public Sector

Overall, private hospitals seem to receive little by way of public subsidies (table 6.8) despite the high profile of the debate over this issue. The practice of public subsidy seems most notable in Uttar Pradesh, where half of large hospitals have received some tax exemptions as nonprofit organizations, and one-third have received discounted land, but few small hospitals in either state have received subsidies.

Compared with other private providers, private hospitals, particularly the big hospitals, had a higher level of current participation in national health programs (table 6.9). Nearly all large hospitals have been involved in polio eradication and the family planning program. However, the desire to participate in national programs was considerably lower in Andhra Pradesh than in Uttar Pradesh. The levels of interest expressed again signal an opportunity for government to work more closely with private hospitals, particularly in Uttar Pradesh.

Table 6.8 Proportion of Private Hospitals that Have Received Public Benefits, Andhra Pradesh and Uttar Pradesh
(percent)

	ANDHRA PRADESH		UTTAR PRADESH	
PUBLIC BENEFIT	SMALL HOSPITALS	LARGE HOSPITALS	SMALL HOSPITALS	LARGE HOSPITALS
Tax exemptions	9	20	9	50
Duty exemptions	1	10	2	25
Reduced utility charges	0	0	0	8
Discounted or free land	1	0	2	33
Low interest loan	4	0	2	0

Note: Small hospitals are those with fewer than 50 beds; large, at least 100 beds.
Source: Background Papers 20 and 21; authors' calculations.

Table 6.9 Participation in National Health Programs by Private Hospitals, Andhra Pradesh and Uttar Pradesh

(percent)

PARTICIPATION	ANDHRA PRADESH		UTTAR PRADESH	
	SMALL HOSPITALS	LARGE HOSPITALS	SMALL HOSPITALS	LARGE HOSPITALS
Desires to participate in national programs	54	40	89	75
Does participate in particular national programs				
Family planning	62	80	53	83
Polio eradication	67	90	80	92
Malaria control	28	50	16	50
Blindness control	25	60	11	58
HIV/AIDS control	42	40	14	50
Tuberculosis control	35	70	30	58
Leprosy control	15	50	11	42

Note: Small hospitals are those with fewer than 50 beds; large, at least 100 beds.
Source: Background Papers 20 and 21; authors' calculations

Concluding Remarks

This chapter revealed new information about the way the private health sector behaves in India, with particular attention given to segments of the market in Andhra Pradesh and Uttar Pradesh. Wide variations were found in the behavior of different market segments and in different geographic areas. Private providers face many obstacles not encountered by the public sector and for the most part have dealt with those obstacles without assistance from government. At the same time, the private sector appears to be interested in working more closely with the public health sector and recognizes the need for greater government oversight and involvement in quality assurance and regulation.

The private sector tends not to measure its performance very closely or to provide much information about its pricing. Otherwise it appears to be more responsive to patient satisfaction than the public sector.

As discussed in part 1, information about the factors that motivate health personnel, transaction costs, the regulatory environment, measurement of performance, and use of partnerships creates options for government intervention. Because the private sector plays such an important role in providing health services and has been ignored by government for so long, a more active and strategic engagement with the private sector should allow it to contribute more fully to improving Indians' health and protecting their financial well-being.

Appendix

Table 6A.1 Distribution of Main Reasons Given by Alternative Private Practitioners in Andhra Pradesh and Uttar Pradesh for Becoming a Medical Practitioner

(percent)

REASON	ANDHRA PRADESH		UTTAR PRADESH	
	UNTRAINED ALLOPATH	NONALLOPATH	UNTRAINED ALLOPATH	NONALLOPATH
Serve people	46	33	48	51
Family tradition or obligation	29	27	12	25
Professional ambition	15	20	8	14
Good income	9	20	32	10
Total	100	100	100	100
Number of providers	85	66	25	59

Note: Andhra Pradesh: chi^2 = 4.75, 3 degrees of freedom; p = 0.2; Uttar Pradesh: chi^2 = 6.98, 3 degrees of freedom; p = 0.07.
Source: Background Papers 20 and 21; authors' calculations.

Table 6A.2 Clinical Conditions Treated by Alternative Private Practitioners over Two Days, Andhra Pradesh and Uttar Pradesh (percent)

	ANDHRA PRADESH			UTTAR PRADESH		
CONDITION TREATED	UNTRAINED ALLOPATH	NON-ALLOPATH	p VALUE	UNTRAINED ALLOPATH	NON-ALLOPATH	p VALUE
Fever	95.6	85.2	0.03	76.0	89.8	0.1
Cough	94.1	94.3	1.0	68.0	81.4	0.2
Pain	92.6	86.4	0.2	80.0	81.4	0.9
Diarrhea	79.4	60.2	0.01	64.0	74.6	0.3
Skin disease	67.6	76.1	0.2	44.0	72.9	0.01
Hypertension	60.3	61.4	0.9	44.0	67.8	0.04
Diabetes	30.9	70.5	<0.001	16.0	39.0	0.03
Tuberculosis	32.4	38.6	0.4	8.0	30.5	0.02
Vaginal discharge	32.4	37.5	0.5	4.0	35.6	0.001
Sexual dysfunction	30.9	39.8	0.2	12.0	44.1	0.03
Penile discharge	29.4	28.4	0.9	8.0	16.9	0.2
Pregnancy-related problem	32.4	23.9	0.2	16.0	22.0	0.5
Insect bite	27.9	27.3	0.9	12.0	3.4	0.2
Fracture	17.6	18.2	0.9	8.0	6.8	0.8
Delivery	19.1	8.0	0.04	4.0	8.5	0.4
Snake bite	16.2	8.0	0.1	4.0	0.0	0.3

Table 6A.3 Patient Fees for an Outpatient Consultation in the Private Sector, Alternative Practitioners Compared with Qualified Allopaths, Andhra Pradesh and Uttar Pradesh

(rupees except as noted)

PROVIDER	ANDHRA PRADESH		UTTAR PRADESH	
	CHARGE	RATIO OF CHARGE TO THAT OF LOWEST-COST PROVIDER	CHARGE	RATIO OF CHARGE TO THAT OF LOWEST-COST PROVIDER
Alternative practitioner				
Untrained allopath	10	1	14	1
Nonallopath	36	3.4	21	1.5
Qualified allopath				
Clinic				
Generalist	33	3.2	66	4.5
Specialist	58	5.6	—	—
Small hospital, outpatient department				
Generalist	45	4.3	54	3.7
Specialist	64	6.1	104	7.2
Large hospital, outpatient department				
Generalist	50	4.8	37	2.6
Specialist	82	7.9	170	11.8

— Not available.
Note: Small hospitals are those with fewer than 50 beds; large, at least 100 beds.
Source: Background Papers 20 and 21; authors' calculations.

Table 6A.4 Allopathic Therapies Offered at Clinics of Alternative Private Practitioners, Andhra Pradesh and Uttar Pradesh
(percent)

	ANDHRA PRADESH			UTTAR PRADESH		
THERAPY	UNTRAINED ALLOPATH	NON-ALLOPATH	p VALUE	UNTRAINED ALLOPATH	NON-ALLOPATH	p VALUE
Paracetemol	84	19	<0.001	92	12	<0.001
Oral antibiotic	79	18	<0.001	76	10	<0.001
Injectable antibiotic	71	11	<0.001	68	10	<0.001
Oral rehydration fluids	68	21	<0.001	64	29	0.003
Intravenous fluids	71	13	<0.001	52	17	0.001
Steroids	25	5	<0.001	32	5	0.002
Oral contraceptives	38	8	<0.001	28	12	0.08
Condoms	28	8	0.001	12	9	0.6
Surgery	10	6	0.3	24	5	0.02

Source: Background Papers 20 and 21; authors' calculations.

Table 6A.5 Concessions Offered to the Poor by Alternative Private Practitioners, Andhra Pradesh and Uttar Pradesh
(percent)

	ANDHRA PRADESH			UTTAR PRADESH		
TYPE OF CONCESSION	UNTRAINED ALLOPATH	NON-ALLOPATH	QUALIFIED ALLOPATHS	UNTRAINED ALLOPATH	NON-ALLOPATH	QUALIFIED ALLOPATHS
Any	99	99	97	100	98	100
Free care	85	84	82	76	93	95
Free samples of medicine	43	59	65	20	22	99
Discount prices	43	33	69	40	44	21
Deferred payment	13	13	35	8	14	1
Less expensive care	9	9	23	12	12	26
Medical camps for poor	4	5	..	12	4	..
Payment in kind	3	6	7	5	0	0

.. Negligible.
Source: Background Papers 20 and 21; authors' calculations.

Table 6A.6 Alternative Private Practitioners Who Rate Government Health Programs as Good or Very Good, Andhra Pradesh and Uttar Pradesh (percent)

PROGRAM	ANDHRA PRADESH		UTTAR PRADESH	
	UNTRAINED ALLOPATH	NONALLOPATH	UNTRAINED ALLOPATH	NONALLOPATH
Family planning	90	78	48	51
Public health	81	75	27	48
Government hospitals	66	61	39	44
Government outpatient services	47	51	22	46

Source: Background Papers 20 and 21; authors' calculations.

Table 6A.7 Private Hospitals Experiencing Moderate or Severe Obstacles to Credit, Andhra Pradesh and Uttar Pradesh (percent)

OBSTACLE	ANDHRA PRADESH		UTTAR PRADESH	
	SMALL HOSPITALS	LARGE HOSPITALS	SMALL HOSPITALS	LARGE HOSPITALS
Too much paperwork for loan	43	25	48	25
Interest rate too high	23	25	40	45
Excessive collateral required	26	25	38	25
Need for connection with bank officials	15	25	32	25
Problems with letters of credit	16	0	14	8
Corruption of bank officials	14	0	5	0
Lack of supplier credits	10	25	12	18
Problems with money transfers	6	25	10	0

Note: Small hospitals are those with fewer than 50 beds; large, at least 100 beds.
Source: Background Papers 20 and 21; authors' calculations.

Table 6A.8 Private Hospitals Making or Planning Capital Investments, Andhra Pradesh and Uttar Pradesh, by Source of Funds
(percent)

INVESTMENT AND SOURCE	ANDHRA PRADESH		UTTAR PRADESH	
	SMALL HOSPITALS	LARGE HOSPITALS	SMALL HOSPITALS	LARGE HOSPITALS
Building investment in past year	32	50	55	75
Bank loan	40	67	33	50
Government	0	0	3	0
Personal resources	50	33	57	25
Donor	5	0	3	25
Equipment investment in past year	57	50	78	92
Bank loan	45	40	57	44
Government	3	0	2	22
Personal resources	56	20	42	0
Donor	6	40	0	33
Capital investment planned	23	10	56	58
Financial partner welcomed	44	0	22	57

Note: Small hospitals are those with fewer than 50 beds; large, at least 100 beds.
Source: Background Papers 20 and 21; authors' calculations.

Table 6A.9 Revenue Issues Affecting Private Hospitals, Andhra Pradesh and Uttar Pradesh
(percent)

REVENUE ISSUE	ANDHRA PRADESH		UTTAR PRADESH	
	SMALL HOSPITALS	LARGE HOSPITALS	SMALL HOSPITALS	LARGE HOSPITALS
Too much competition from other hospitals	64	38	60	36
Nonpayment by patients	65	33	36	25
Too few paying patients	27	22	40	27
Nonpayment by government	7	0	16	30
Nonpayment by employers under contract	19	17	8	11
Donations reduced	2	0	2	0
Revenues exceeding operating expenses	87	88	91	92
Income rising	77	86	79	83

Note: Small hospitals are those with fewer than 50 beds; large, at least 100 beds.
Source: Background Papers 20 and 21; authors' calculations.

Table 6A.10 Labor Issues in Private Hospitals, Andhra Pradesh and Uttar Pradesh

(percent)

ISSUE	ANDHRA PRADESH		UTTAR PRADESH	
	SMALL HOSPITALS	LARGE HOSPITALS	SMALL HOSPITALS	LARGE HOSPITALS
Low productivity of labor	41	33	48	25
High cost of skilled employees	27	50	45	17
Scarcity of skilled employees	40	33	48	27
Missed work due to illness	17	50	18	0
Absenteeism	34	33	19	17
Lack of skilled management	24	33	13	0
Regulations on working conditions	14	33	19	8
Restrictions on laying off workers	12	17	10	0
High staff turnover	11	33	14	0
Union activities/restrictions	6	17	2	0
Seasonal shortages of unskilled labor	9	0	8	8

Note: Small hospitals are those with fewer than 50 beds; large, at least 100 beds.
Source: Background Papers 20 and 21 and authors' calculations.

Table 6A.11 Public Infrastructure Issues Affecting Private Hospitals, Andhra Pradesh and Uttar Pradesh

(percent)

ISSUE	ANDHRA PRADESH		UTTAR PRADESH	
	SMALL HOSPITALS	LARGE HOSPITALS	SMALL HOSPITALS	LARGE HOSPITALS
Electricity breakdowns	62	50	94	83
Poor drainage	45	50	72	55
Telecommunications breakdowns	45	25	63	67
Inadequate water supply	39	53	64	33
General waste disposal problems	25	25	63	50
Biomedical waste disposal problems	23	13	61	50
Availability of transportation	23	0	27	0
Access to land	22	25	21	9
Availability of office space	22	0	12	0

Note: Small hospitals are those with fewer than 50 beds; large, at least 100 beds.
Source: Background Papers 20 and 21; authors' calculations.

Table 6A.12 Regulatory Issues Affecting Hospital Managers, Andhra Pradesh and Uttar Pradesh
(percent)

ISSUE	ANDHRA PRADESH		UTTAR PRADESH	
	SMALL HOSPITALS	LARGE HOSPITALS	SMALL HOSPITALS	LARGE HOSPITALS
High taxes	26	40	76	50
Judicial system	14	40	66	50
Tax administration	15	20	59	42
Government clearances	22	40	57	64
Unfair competition from other providers	20	60	46	42
Government official corruption	20	40	46	50
Police corruption	14	20	40	42
Labor union regulation	12	50	39	40
Quality standards	18	20	24	17
Price controls	8	0	33	25

Note: Small hospitals are those with fewer than 50 beds; large, at least 100 beds.
Source: Background Papers 20 and 21; authors' calculations.

Table 6A.13 Ideal Job Characteristics Reported by Public and Private Sector Health Workers, Andhra Pradesh and Uttar Pradesh (percent)

JOB CHARACTERISTIC	ANDHRA PRADESH		UTTAR PRADESH	
	PUBLIC SECTOR	PRIVATE SECTOR	PUBLIC SECTOR	PRIVATE SECTOR
Work environment				
Good physical working conditions	90.9	90.5	91.7	94.2
Knowing what you are expected to do and achieve at work	83.8	72.2	90.5	89.6
Freedom from political interference in decisionmaking	80.6	79.5	76.9	85.9
Not needing to pay bribes to get what you want	73.1	75.9	87.7	87.9
Knowing you can keep your job as long as you want	57.8	52.9	69.1	73.3
Professional fulfillment				
Training opportunities to improve skills or learn new skills	90.5	82.5	94.2	93.4
Challenging work that offers a sense of accomplishment	88.8	84.4	91.5	91.5
Tools and materials to use skills fully on the job	83.0	84.4	95.7	93.0
Good opportunities to advance to a better job	75.1	64.1	94.6	77.7
Work relationships				
Good working relationship with colleagues	93.8	91.0	98.2	97.8
Superior recognizes good work	74.7	62.6	93.6	68.8
Respected and trusted by clients	69.7	74.5	94.1	93.2
Independence from interference by superiors	59.2	50.7	54.7	61.6
Personal benefits				
Desirable location (e.g., one with good schools)	83.5	73.6	93.9	84.3
Sufficient time for personal or family life	78.5	75.7	93.7	85.5
Good employment benefits (e.g., pension, housing)	78.5	54.8	93.9	65.8
Good income	76.3	66.2	84.6	73.4

Source: Background Papers 20 and 21; STEM (2000).

Table 6A.14 Presence in Current Job of Ideal Job Characteristics, as Reported by Public and Private Health Sector Workers, Andhra Pradesh and Uttar Pradesh (percent)

JOB CHARACTERISTIC	ANDHRA PRADESH		UTTAR PRADESH	
	PUBLIC SECTOR	PRIVATE SECTOR	PUBLIC SECTOR	PRIVATE SECTOR
Work environment				
Good physical working conditions	53.3	61.1	42.6	78.9
Knowing what you are expected to do and achieve at work	61.8	61.6	64.3	79.5
Freedom from political interference in decisionmaking	69.3	79.4	35.3	89.9
Not needing to pay bribes to get what you want	69.9	74.6	15.3	89.1
Knowing you can keep your job as long as you want	44.5	50.4	48.2	71.1
Professional fulfillment				
Training opportunities to improve skills or learn new skills	42.9	29.9	21.7	49.0
Challenging work that offers a sense of accomplishment	61.6	62.1	51.8	74.0
Tools and materials to use skills fully on the job	35.5	52.3	40.1	75.5
Good opportunities to advance to a better job	37.1	33.9	30.7	41.4
Work relationships				
Good working relationship with colleagues	83.5	79.5	80.5	90.1
Superior recognizes good work	50.8	44.2	55.5	43.4
Respected and trusted by clients	57.3	67.4	76.0	91.5
Independence from interference by superiors	39.4	39.8	38.5	49.9
Personal benefits				
Desirable location (e.g., one with good schools)	51.0	53.6	36.7	78.7
Sufficient time for personal or family life	35.7	36.0	50.0	55.0
Good employment benefits (e.g., pension, housing)	45.8	23.4	42.7	22.2
Good income	36.1	38.1	42.8	45.2

Source: Background Papers 20 and 21; STEM (2000).

Table 6A.15 Presence of Ideal Job Characteristics in Andhra Pradesh: Differences in Ratings between Public and Private Sector, by Characteristic of Health Worker

JOB CHARACTERISTIC	CHARACTERISTIC OF HEALTH WORKER THAT PREDICTED SIGNIFICANTLY HIGHER RATINGS OF PRESENCE OF JOB CHARACTERISTIC
Work environment	
Good physical working conditions	Private sector; small hospitals; specialists
Freedom from political interference in decisionmaking	Private sector; specialist and general doctors
Professional fulfillment	
Tools and materials to use skills fully on the job	Private sector; small hospitals; specialist and general doctors; males
Work relationships	
Superior recognizes good work	Public sector; nurses; younger age
Respected and trusted by clients	Private sector; clinics or primary health centers; males
Personal benefits	
Desirable location (e.g., one with good schools)	Private sector
Good employment benefits (e.g., pension, housing)	Public sector
Good income	Private sector; large hospitals; specialist and general doctors; males

Note: Multivariate models are built as follows: Motivating factor = $b_{intercept}$ + b_{public} + $b_{profession}$ + $b_{facility\ size}$ + b_{sex} + b_{age} + error. The comparison group for profession is nurses (versus specialists and general allopaths), and for facility is clinics (versus small hospitals, large hospitals, and diagnostic centers). Characteristics are ordered from largest to smallest proportion of variance explained in the model. Small hospitals are those with fewer than 50 beds; large, at least 100 beds.

Table 6A.16 Average Number of Full-Time and Part-Time Nurses and Private and Government Doctors Working in Private Hospitals, Andhra Pradesh and Uttar Pradesh

	ANDHRA PRADESH		UTTAR PRADESH	
PRACTITIONER	PUBLIC SECTOR	PRIVATE SECTOR	PUBLIC SECTOR	PRIVATE SECTOR
Certified nurses				
Full time	2.1	20.2	7.0	27.1
Part time	0.1	0.0	0.1	0.0
Private doctors				
Specialists				
Full time	1.3	8.0	2.4	17.9
Part time	1.4	6.4	3.6	9.1
Generalists				
Full time	0.9	7.7	0.9	3.7
Part time	0.1	0.0	0.2	0.0
Government doctors, part time				
Specialists	0.6	8.0	0.2	1.0
Generalists	0.0	0.0	0.0	0.0

Note: Small hospitals are those with fewer than 50 beds; large, at least 100 beds.
Source: Background Papers 20 and 21; authors' calculations.

Notes

1.   The two types of providers were combined because they were sampled together and later distinguished based on their answers in the questionnaires; allopaths were given a different questionnaire.

2.   Patient exit interviews come from both outpatients and inpatients at hospitals.

3.   The researchers were unable to distinguish the results of those who practice in both the public and private sectors, as respondents were categorized according to their work location.

4. No universal agreement exists as to the optimal cesarean section rate, but some authors have argued that a rate of about 6 percent to 8 percent would be an appropriate response to the common medical indications for the surgery (Francome and Savage 1993). During a consensus-building exercise by the World Health Organization, a rate of 10–15 percent was considered appropriate (WHO 1985), although the rate was defined somewhat arbitrarily. The U.S. government, in its *Healthy People 2000* strategy, set a goal of reducing the cesarean section rate to 15 percent by 2000 (U.S. Department of Health and Human Services 1991). Where the population is impoverished and general and reproductive health are poor (conditions leading to high-risk pregnancies), some have argued that a rate of 20 percent may be appropriate.

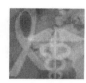

CHAPTER 7

Setting National Health Care Priorities and Ensuring Equitable Delivery of Public Sector Services

This chapter considers four aspects of public health care spending: (a) the extent to which centrally sponsored schemes meet India's health care needs, (b) the division of service utilization between the public and private sectors, (c) the degree of equity in current public health care spending, and (d) the implications of current patterns of public health care spending for health outcomes (see box 7.1 for a summary of the empirical findings and policy challenges discussed in the chapter).

Do Centrally Sponsored Schemes Meet India's Health Care Needs?

National priority programs, or centrally sponsored schemes, have traditionally been justified on one or more of the following grounds: they provide a public good; significant externalities exist; the magnitude of the health problem is enormous; beneficiaries are predominantly poor; and affordable, effective intervention is available. The health issues addressed by these programs have been deemed to be of national importance. Rapid population growth and the emerging

Box 7.1 Empirical Findings and Policy Challenges

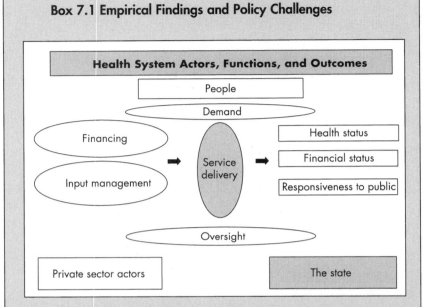

Health System Actors, Functions, and Outcomes

People

Demand

Financing

Health status

Service delivery

Financial status

Input management

Responsiveness to public

Oversight

Private sector actors

The state

Empirical Findings

- National programs continue to address much of the disease burden in India.
- As India's disease profile changes, important public health problems, including cardiovascular disease, mental illness, injury prevention, and the risks associated with tobacco, will need to be addressed.
- The poor in India smoke more and use nonsmoking tobacco and alcohol more than the population as a whole, placing them at higher risk for developing certain noncommunicable diseases.

Findings from the analysis of household data from the 52nd round of the National Sample Survey:

National Level

- The private sector accounts for 82 percent of outpatient care, 56 percent of hospitalizations, 46 percent of institutional deliveries, and 40 percent of prenatal care visits. It provides only 10 percent of immunizations.
- As in most developing countries, richer households purchase more curative health care from the private sector than do poorer households.
- Public spending on curative services is highly pro-rich: nationwide Rs 3 is spent on the richest 20 percent for every Rs 1 spent on the poorest 20 percent.
- The distribution of public outpatient services are pro-poor, particularly at the primary health center level. Inpatient services are less likely than outpatient services to reach the poor.
- The public sector provides most health services to Indians living below the poverty line, accounting for 93 percent of immunizations, 74 of prenatal care, 69 percent of institutional deliveries, and 60 percent of hospitalizations. The exception is outpatient care, where the private sector accounts for 79 percent of the care for the poor.

Regional Level

- The use of public services is more equitable in urban areas than in rural areas.
- In Kerala, Tamil Nadu, and Maharashtra, the distribution of public spending on health is nearly uniform across income groups. In six states, however, more than Rs 4 goes to the richest quintile for every Rs 1 that reaches the poorest.
- Health status outcomes are better in states in which public spending on health care is more equitable.

Box 7.1 (continued)

Policy Challenges

- How can implementation of national public health programs be strengthened by addressing critical gaps in program management, technical leadership, and communication?
- How and when should effective programs that address emerging public health problems—cardiovascular disease, mental illness, injuries, and the health consequences of smoking—be developed?
- How can the distribution of public spending be improved so that a greater share of spending reaches the poor?
- How can the quality and accountability of public and private health services be improved?

HIV/AIDS epidemic, for example, pose significant threats to India's future economic and social prospects. Widespread health problems with significant externalities are addressed by programs of disease control, such as those for tuberculosis, leprosy, and malaria, and by safe motherhood and child health interventions such as immunizations. Curing one case of tuberculosis, for example, can prevent the spread of infection to as many as 15 people (WHO 2000a). Iodizing salt and draining swamps for malaria control are public goods whose benefits are shared across the population. Integrated Child Development Services, a program that addresses malnutrition, is intended to target benefits to the poor.

Many national programs have received additional support in recent years because they have introduced new cost-effective technologies. Intraocular lenses are now implanted as part of blindness control. Tuberculosis control now uses directly observed treatment, short courses. Multidrug therapy is used for leprosy control, and a new mix of case management and prevention techniques is used to control malaria.

In 1990, centrally sponsored schemes addressed conditions affecting more than 40 percent of the deaths and 46 percent of the DALYs lost in India.[1] By 1998 the number of deaths and DALYs lost associated with these conditions had fallen 15 percent, but they still accounted for 34 percent of all deaths and 42 percent of DALYs lost (table 7.1).

Most centrally sponsored programs are available to all Indians, but the programs are expected to ensure that basic services are available to the poor. Program activities for leprosy control and malaria control target the poorest states and they also target the poorest districts within states in which these diseases are most prevalent. These programs increase the welfare of the poor. An analysis of employability and earnings of people with leprosy in Tamil Nadu, for example, found that eliminating the deformity would raise the probability of gainful employment from 42 percent to 78 percent and increase the annual earnings per employed person 119 percent (World Bank 2001). The combined effect of increased employment and increased earnings would triple the annual earnings of all people with leprosy.

The large burden of disease, large externalities, poverty dimensions, and cost-effectiveness of the interventions covered by the current national priority programs suggest that they remain a good fit for public intervention. The main challenge is improving their implementation.

Because India's disease profile is changing, several major health conditions that account for a large burden of disease are not covered under current national health programs (table 7.2). The proportion of deaths associated with tobacco use, for example, rose to more than 25 percent in 1998 (risk factors other than tobacco use contribute to these diseases as well). Since these conditions largely affect older people, they represent a much smaller, albeit still significant, burden of DALYs lost (8 percent). Major psychiatric diseases (unipolar and bipolar disease, psychoses, self-inflicted injuries) account for 6.6 percent of DALYs lost— more than either tuberculosis or HIV. Injuries, particularly from traffic accidents, fires, and falls, also represent a large (8.9 percent) and

Table 7.1 Deaths and DALYs Lost Associated with Conditions Covered by National Health Programs, India, 1990 and 1998

PROGRAM	DEATHS				DALYS LOST			
	1990		1998		1990		1998	
	NUMBER (THOUSANDS)	PERCENT OF TOTAL	NUMBER (THOUSANDS)	PERCENT OF TOTAL	NUMBER (THOUSANDS)	PERCENT OF TOTAL	NUMBER (THOUSANDS)	PERCENT OF TOTAL
Reproductive and child health	2,962	31.6	2,492	26.7	109,955	38.2	91,431	34.0
Safe motherhood	775	8.3	737	7.9	32,772	11.4	31,207	11.6
Immunization	513	5.5	429	4.6	18,328	6.4	14,463	5.4
Control of diarrhea, disease, and acute respiratory infections	1,624	17.3	1,285	13.8	52,124	18.1	38,893	14.5
Vitamin A supplementation	21	0.2	16	0.2	746	0.3	565	0.2
Anemia control	29	0.3	26	0.3	5,985	2.1	6,302	2.3
Integrated Child Development Services	69	0.7	53	0.6	5,076	1.8	3,734	1.4
Protein energy malnutrition	69	0.7	53	0.6	5,076	1.8	3,734	1.4
Universal salt iodization	6	0.1	5	..	378	0.1	280	0.1
Communicable disease control	780	8.3	621	6.6	15,380	5.3	13,973	5.2
Tuberculosis control	752	8.0	421	4.5	13,763	4.8	7,577	2.8
HIV/AIDS control	1	..	179	1.9	236	0.1	5,611	2.1
Malaria control	26	0.3	20	0.2	1,195	0.4	577	0.2
Leprosy	1	..	1	..	186	0.1	208	0.1
Blindness control	0	..	0	..	3,038	1.1	3,732	1.4
Total national programs	3,811	40.7	3,166	33.9	133,449	46.4	112,869	42.0
Total	9,371	100	9,337	100	287,739	100	268,953	100

.. Negligible.
Source: Murray and Lopez (1996); WHO (1999).

Table 7.2 Deaths and DALYs Lost Associated with Major Conditions Not Covered by National Health Programs, India, 1990 and 1998

PROGRAM	DEATHS				DALYS LOST			
	1990		1998		1990		1998	
	NUMBER (THOUSANDS)	PERCENT OF TOTAL	NUMBER (THOUSANDS)	PERCENT OF TOTAL	NUMBER (THOUSANDS)	PERCENT OF TOTAL	NUMBER (THOUSANDS)	PERCENT OF TOTAL
Respiratory and circulatory illnesses	1,878	20.0	2,360	25.3	18,347	6.4	21,282	7.9
Trachea, bronchus, lung neoplasm	35	0.4	79	0.8	387	0.1	921	0.3
Mouth and oropharynx cancers	80	0.9	100	1.1	1,100	0.4	1,313	0.5
Ischemic heart disease	1,175	12.5	1 471	15.8	10,131	3.5	11,697	4.3
Cerebrovascular disease	448	4.8	557	6.0	4,235	1.5	4,814	1.8
Chronic obstructive pulmonary disease	140	1.5	153	1.6	2,494	0.9	2,536	0.9
Mental health	107	1.2	7	1.4	14,821	5.2	17,726	6.6
Unipolar major depression	1	..	0	..	8,063	2.8	9,679	3.6
Bipolar affective disorder	2	..	2	..	2,305	0.8	2,746	1.0
Psychoses	5	0.1	5	0.1	1,650	0.6	1,964	0.7
Self-inflicted injury	99	1.1	124	1.3	3,337	1.2	3,337	1.2
Injuries	344	3.7	401	4.3	21,821	7.6	23,824	8.9
Road traffic injuries	174	1.9	217	2.3	5,992	2.1	7,204	2.7
Fire	124	1.3	135	1.4	5,647	2.0	5,723	2.1
Falls	46	0.5	50	0.5	10,182	3.5	10,898	4.1

.. Negligible.
Source: Murray and Lopez (1996); WHO (1999).

growing share of India's burden of disease. Violence against women has been neglected in India and many other countries, though new approaches are being developed to deal with these situations (box 7.2).

Prevention of tobacco-related disease is a classic public health issue for which a mix of social marketing activities (such as education and publicity) and regulation is appropriate. International estimates suggest that tobacco control interventions cost $20–$80 per DALY saved (World Bank 1999a), a reasonable level of cost-effectiveness. Whether cost-effective interventions can be provided in India for tobacco-related diseases and the other problems not covered by national programs depends to a large extent on the implementation capacity of the agencies involved.[2]

The poverty dimension to noncommunicable diseases is often overlooked in low-income countries. Such diseases become more prominent as mortality levels fall and national incomes increase; as countries undergo a health transition, the burden of such ailments is sometimes assumed to fall disproportionately on the higher social classes. The scant data available in India, however, suggest that people in rural Rajasthan with low education levels and unskilled jobs are already suffering higher rates of coronary heart disease and hypertension than the more educated and skilled (Gupta, Gupta, and Ahluwalia 1994). Analysis of risk factors for cardiovascular disease shows that tobacco use is higher among illiterate men and unskilled workers in urban and rural settings in India than among the literate and more skilled (Gupta, Gupta, and Ahluwalia 1994; Reddy and others 2000; Prabhakaran and others 2000). National Sample Survey data show that throughout India the prevalence of tobacco and alcohol use is higher among the poor than among the nonpoor, which puts the risk of cardiovascular disease among the poor, other things being equal, at a higher level than it is for others (figure 7.1). In turn, these higher risks may lead to higher rates of cardiovascular disease, cancer, liver disease, and injuries among the poor than among the nonpoor.

The degree to which programs addressing serious mental conditions affect the poor has not been well studied in India. In other countries the poor and the most vulnerable are more likely to be

Box 7.2 Responding to Violence against Women

In Mumbai, a city of 14 million people, the Bombay Municipal Corporation (BMC) manages a network of 26 hospitals with a staff 17,000 health workers. In two of its hospitals located in the poorer sections of the city, the BMC is piloting One Stop Crisis Centers to assist women injured by domestic and sexual violence.

In addition to providing medical and psychological care, the One Stop Crisis Centers will consolidate in one place key related services offered by other agencies such as the police, the welfare department, legal aid, and shelters. The hospitals' Emergency Department would run the center and be responsible for establishing links with the other agencies.

The initiative is a collaboration among the BMC, an NGO (Center for Enquiry into Health and Allied Themes [CEHAT]), and the Ford Foundation. CEHAT is training the BMC staff who will run the center. It is also providing support for two experts to be located at the center for its first two years for supervising, coordinating with other agencies, and setting up systems. The project includes a research component to document the prevalence of domestic and sexual violence and develop new forms for record taking.

BMC and CEHAT designed the One Stop Crisis Center concept on the basis of lessons learned from similar crisis centers established extensively in hospitals in Malaysia and the Philippines. Some key lessons incorporated into the Mumbai design are that:

- The hospital is a good venue for providing crisis center services.
- Government agencies and NGOs can work together effectively on targeted interventions.
- Through community outreach, crisis centers can provide prevention as well as treatment programs.

The need for One Stop Crisis Centers is large, and the BMC is seeking to implement a low-cost model that can be replicated in other hospitals.

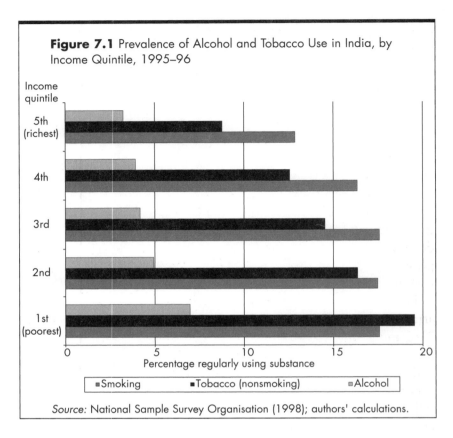

Figure 7.1 Prevalence of Alcohol and Tobacco Use in India, by Income Quintile, 1995–96

Source: National Sample Survey Organisation (1998); authors' calculations.

affected by serious mental conditions (Dohrenwend and Dohrenwend 1969), and major depression has been linked to loss of employability (Eaton, Day, and Kramer 1988). In India, major psychosis is likely to be most common among the most destitute of people.

Treatment of affective disorders and psychosis involves supervised community outreach workers, pharmaceuticals, and structured programs to keep people living safely and working in their communities. Like other disease control programs, these programs rely on an effective referral system. No estimates exist of the feasibility of such treatment in India or of their cost-effectiveness. Studies conducted in other parts of the world have estimated the cost of community-based mental health programs at $250–$999 per DALY saved

(World Bank 1993), making these programs much more cost-effective than most hospital-based interventions.

The government may also have to consider providing support to other types of programs that the private sector is unlikely to finance. These include interventions whose effectiveness and efficiency are difficult to quantify but that are nevertheless important to India's health system. Examples include public education on health, health information systems, disease surveillance, pharmaceutical quality control, and other types of regulatory interventions.

In addition to determining which kinds of programs to offer, policymakers need to decide how best to implement programs. Should government provide services directly, finance them, or both? As we document below, the vast majority of outpatient visits are to private providers; can centrally sponsored programs work more effectively with the private sector?

For services the public sector provides, what type of institutional arrangements are most effective? Spurred in part by the passage of the 73rd and 74th Amendments to the Constitution, administrators are increasingly devolving the management of health programs to state and local bodies. The current dilemma is that the central government is not able to manage centrally sponsored programs without greater reliance on the states and local bodies, but states and local bodies have little capacity to manage these programs themselves.

Recent reviews of the Reproductive and Child Health Program and other centrally sponsored programs have suggested that India continues to suffer from critical gaps in its capacity for planning, implementing, and monitoring the outcomes of these programs. Many of the difficulties are tied to underlying weaknesses of the general health systems on which these programs depend. Shortages exist in technical leadership, public health management, and the capacity to plan and manage public communications. The hierarchical administrative processes at the central and state levels continue under the guise of financial and administrative accountability, lengthening delays in implementation and weakening the responsiveness of programs to local needs.

Interestingly, when states are given more flexibility, many prefer not to exercise it fully. Under the Reproductive and Child Health Program, for example, the Ministry of Health and Family Welfare has offered to decentralize procurement, but so far only one state (Tamil Nadu) has responded. What's needed is more accountability for program outputs and outcomes, but the emphasis is often on administering inputs and expenditures. The current challenge is to address the increasing need to decentralize and integrate health programs while strengthening skills, creating systems, and building local demand. For some programs, separate program management and financing will remain the best alternative. Examination of the motivation and behavior of workers in the public health sector may also provide insights about alternative ways of providing or financing health interventions, a subject explored in the next chapter.

Households' Use of Personal Health Services

Unlike the use of community-based public health services, which is driven by government, the use of personal health services is determined by individuals and households. People choose whether or not to seek out medical care, which type of providers to consult (and in what order), and whether to comply with the recommended therapy. These choices are constrained, especially for the poor, by lack of income, time, knowledge of the disease, and information about the efficacy of various types of providers. This section examines how these choices affect the pattern of consumption of health services provided by the public and private sectors.

National Findings

As noted in the preceding chapter, the distribution of consumption of services provided by the public and private sectors varies by type of service (figure 6.1). The National Sample Survey data distinguish five types of services: outpatient care, inpatient care (excluding deliveries),

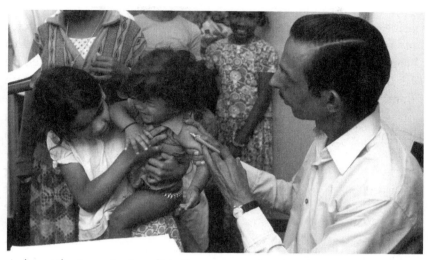

A day at the immunization clinic (PHOTOGRAPH BY RAY WITLIN/THE WORLD BANK PHOTO LIBRARY)

institutional deliveries, prenatal care, and immunizations. Outpatient care is dominated by the private sector, which accounts for 83 percent of all outpatient visits. Hospitalizations and institutional deliveries are split about equally between the public and private sectors. The public sector plays the larger role in preventive services, delivering 60 percent of prenatal visits and 90 percent of immunization doses.

The high percentage of outpatient services provided by the private sector is similar across household income and expenditure levels, urban and rural settings, gender, and caste and tribe affiliation. The poor do, however, use a different class of provider than do the rich, with the poor relying more on untrained practitioners and the rich using qualified practitioners.

Both public and private hospitalizations increase with income (figure 7.2). Relative to people in the bottom income quintile, people in the top income quintile have almost six times as many hospitalizations—about twice as many hospitalizations in the public sector and about 11 times as many private hospitalizations.

The poor depend on public hospitals more than the rich; for the poorest quintiles, 61 percent of hospitalizations are in public hospi-

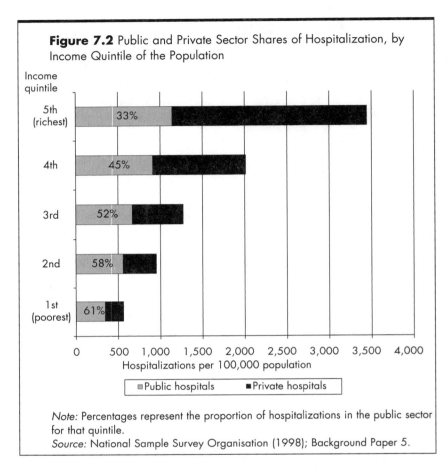

Figure 7.2 Public and Private Sector Shares of Hospitalization, by Income Quintile of the Population

Note: Percentages represent the proportion of hospitalizations in the public sector for that quintile.
Source: National Sample Survey Organisation (1998); Background Paper 5.

tals. However, even those in the poorest quintile of the population use the private sector for nearly 40 percent of hospitalizations, even though the reported hospital charges per inpatient day are eight times higher in the private sector (Rs 48 per day in private facilities versus Rs 6 per day in public facilities).

Institutional deliveries reveal a similar pattern. Individuals in the top income quintile are three times more likely to use the public sector for institutional deliveries than the poorest quintile and 20 times more likely to use the private sector. Poor women who deliver in an institution are most likely to do so in public facilities, which account for 73 percent of institutional deliveries among women in the bottom income quintile.

An important dimension to hospitalization is the length of stay (number of inpatient bed days). Long-term hospitalizations of the rich account for a large proportion of hospital days in the public sector. Stays of more than 90 days account for more than one-fourth of all public inpatient bed days, and 40 percent of those stays are by the richest quintile. The fact that the rich account for a disproportionate share of inpatient bed days raises questions about the need for appropriate policies to improve equity and efficiency. For example, a long-term care policy may include higher fees for richer Indians having long-term stays or the establishment of a different level of facility to keep costs down.

As with the income quintile findings, people below the poverty line are more likely than people above the poverty line to use the public sector. Two types of services—inpatient bed days and prenatal care—show the greatest variation. For people living below the poverty line, 66 percent of inpatient bed days take place in public facilities; for people living above the poverty line, only 44 percent of bed days are in public facilities. Similarly, 74 percent of prenatal visits by women below the poverty line take place in public facilities, while only 52 percent of visits by women above the poverty line are provided by the public sector.

A striking finding of the National Sample Survey is the gross underutilization of inpatient beds at primary health care facilities. While an estimated 20 percent of all public sector inpatient beds in India are at primary health centers, less than 5 percent of inpatient bed days take place at these centers. Moreover, these centers are not particularly pro-poor. The inability of these facilities to provide staff and ensure supplies contributes to their low quality and utilization (Mukhopadhyay 1997). Exercises conducted as part of State Health Systems Development Projects to rationalize public health services and design referral systems have shown that inpatient beds at primary health facilities are not needed, suggesting that the government should no longer invest in these beds. In states in which budgets are allocated on the basis of the number of beds, the budget allocation practice would have to be changed.

State-Level Findings

The distribution between private and public provision of personal health services varies considerably across states. To simplify the presentation, we discuss only inpatient curative care and institutional delivery services here. Inpatient curative care is included because hospitalization accounts for the largest outlay of both public and private resources; institutional deliveries are included because they are a determinant and leading indicator of maternal illness and death.

National data show a relatively even distribution of inpatient bed days between the public and private sectors. State data show much greater variation. The use of public hospitals is much higher than average in several states, including Himachal Pradesh (92 percent), Orissa (89 percent), West Bengal (81 percent), the Northeast states (77 percent), and Rajasthan (74 percent). Elsewhere—in Haryana (24 percent), Punjab (34 percent), and Maharashtra (36 percent)— the use of public facilities is lower than average.

Large variations across states are also evident in the use of public versus private facilities by those below the poverty line (figure 7.3). In West Bengal and Orissa, the poor are heavy users of public facilities. In contrast, the poor in Punjab and Bihar make very limited use of the public sector.

The use of public and private facilities for institutional deliveries also differs across states. Nationwide, the public sector share of bed days for deliveries is 50 percent. Utilization of public facilities is significantly higher than the national average in Orissa (89 percent), Uttar Pradesh (81 percent), and the Northeastern states (77 percent). States exhibiting less reliance on the public sector include Haryana (24 percent), Punjab (34 percent), and Maharashtra (36 percent). The same basic distribution between public and private facilities across states appears among women living below the poverty line.

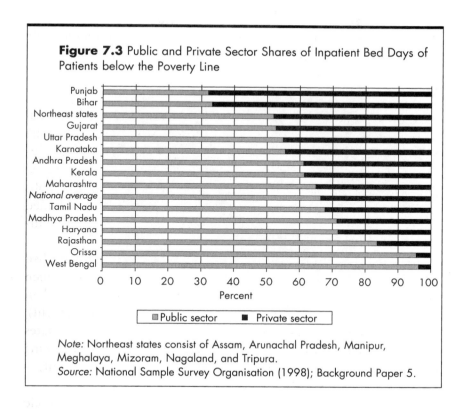

Figure 7.3 Public and Private Sector Shares of Inpatient Bed Days of Patients below the Poverty Line

Note: Northeast states consist of Assam, Arunachal Pradesh, Manipur, Meghalaya, Mizoram, Nagaland, and Tripura.
Source: National Sample Survey Organisation (1998); Background Paper 5.

How Well Are Public Health Services Reaching the Poor?

In the historical context of building a socialist nation, India's early plans for a public national health service that would provide services to all—a system similar to that being created simultaneously in the United Kingdom—were easy to justify. Public funds sufficient to maintain such a comprehensive health care system were never forthcoming, however. In the absence of an adequate public system, the private sector has grown dramatically. By the time of the National Health Policy in 1983, the concern for equity—particularly the need to provide health services to the poor—had become the main rhetorical justification for publicly provided curative health services. (The other rationale was the need to train doctors and other medical professions. This rationale is the foundation for public involvement in tertiary health care.) India's Constitution laid most of the responsibility for providing curative care in the hands of the states.[3]

The analysis presented here estimates the relative size of the financial subsidy provided to people at different income or expenditure levels through government health care services. It is based on data from the study on the benefit incidence of health services (Background Paper 5), which in turn derived its information from budget and cost data for public health services and data from the 52nd round of the National Sample Survey (1995–96), which covered more than 121,000 households.[4]

National Findings

For the nation as a whole, the poorest 20 percent of the population captured only about 10 percent of the total net public subsidy from publicly provided clinical services (figure 7.4). The richest quintile received more than the three times the subsidy received by the poorest quintile, indicating that publicly financed curative care services are unambiguously pro-rich. In part, this bias reflects the fact that the better-off use public facilities more than the poor, but it also reflects the fact that they pay more than the poor for each unit of utilization. For example, the top two quintiles (the richest 40 percent) pay 87.6 percent of the collected fees for inpatient care.

The better-off pay higher fees because they receive higher-quality service—a fact not captured by the benefit incidence data. Net cost recovery (fees relative to incremental costs of services) may therefore well differ from that implied by the amounts presented. Moreover, except in three states, cost recovery is low, with fees never exceeding 5 percent of costs. These amounts suggest that a better system for ensuring that the poor receive at least their fair share of public health expenditures needs to be put in place.

An alternative approach to assessing the distributional performance of the health sector is to use poverty measures based on a poverty line for rural and urban areas in each state. This approach

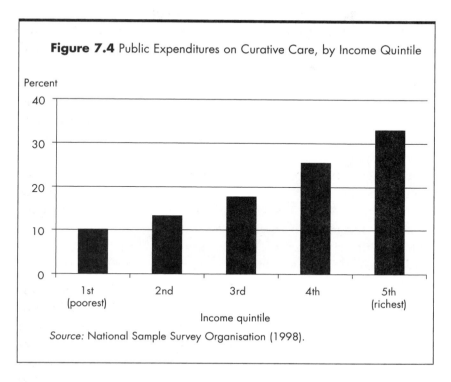

Figure 7.4 Public Expenditures on Curative Care, by Income Quintile

Percent

Source: National Sample Survey Organisation (1998).

reveals that while 36 percent of the nation's people live below the poverty line, they receive only about 24 percent of public financing of curative health services.[5]

The pro-rich distribution of public health care expenditures in India reflects several factors:

- For a given health condition, the rich are more likely to seek care, and when they do they are more likely to go to a higher-level facility. The richest quintile of the population is thus six times more likely than the poorest quintile to have been hospitalized in either the public or private sector (3,447 versus 563 per 100,000).

- The richest quintile accounts for 38.5 percent of inpatient bed days, while the poorest quintile accounts for just 6.6 percent.

- Because hospital costs represent by far the largest share of curative health costs (87 percent) and curative health costs dominate aggregate health care spending, aggregate health expenditures are dominated by hospital expenditures.[6]

The health care spending gap between rich and poor is even wider in the private sector. Thus, without public sector spending, the gap between rich and poor in service utilization would be even larger. Private sector facilities accounted for 67 percent of hospitals visits by the richest quintile. For the poorest quintile, such facilities accounted for 39 percent of hospital visits.

The pro-rich bias varies across categories and types of health spending (figure 7.5). A concentration curve below the diagonal line indicates that the rich receive a more than proportional share of public health spending; a concentration curve above the diagonal line indicates a pro-poor bias. Outpatient care in primary care facilities shows a slight pro-poor bias, while spending on both inpatient and outpatient hospital care is biased toward the rich.

Preventive care, immunizations, and prenatal visits show a more equitable distribution than most types of curative care. The public subsidy for immunizations is pro-poor, with the poorest two quintiles receiving 47 percent of all publicly provided doses (figure 7.6). Some, but not all, of the pro-poor distribution can be explained by the fact that poor households have more children. Prenatal care services provided at primary care facilities also appear to be pro-poor, with the bottom two quintiles accounting for 46 percent of visits.

A major limitation of the National Sample Survey data is that they do not allow deeper exploration of hospital-based services. The data do not distinguish between large urban tertiary hospitals and small rural secondary hospitals. A recent summary of international evidence argues that the poor are more likely to use primary care facilities than secondary care facilities, and more likely to use secondary care facilities than tertiary facilities (Yaqub 1999). Moreover, analysis of facility-based data in several Indian states shows that the poor use proportionately more secondary hospitals, particularly those located in poorer rural areas (STEM 2000; Institute of Health Systems 2000; Blackstone Ltd. 2000). This may mean that the use of

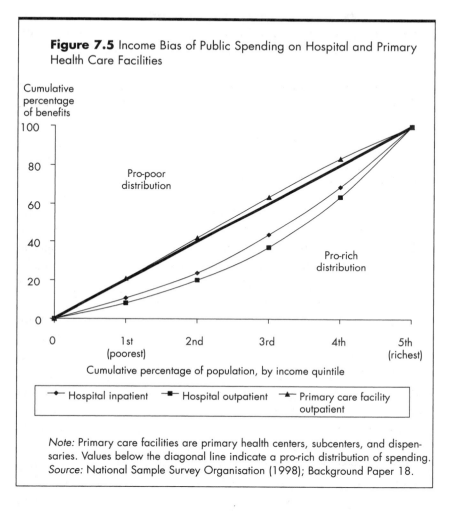

Figure 7.5 Income Bias of Public Spending on Hospital and Primary Health Care Facilities

Cumulative percentage of benefits

Pro-poor distribution

Pro-rich distribution

Cumulative percentage of population, by income quintile

0   1st (poorest)   2nd   3rd   4th   5th (richest)

—◆— Hospital inpatient   —■— Hospital outpatient   —▲— Primary care facility outpatient

Note: Primary care facilities are primary health centers, subcenters, and dispensaries. Values below the diagonal line indicate a pro-rich distribution of spending.
Source: National Sample Survey Organisation (1998); Background Paper 18.

secondary hospitals is not as pro-rich as that of all hospitals taken together.

Segmenting the data by region shows that rural residents receive a lower public subsidy than urban residents: although 75 percent of India's population live in rural areas, rural residents capture only 67.6 percent of the net benefits from curative care. The concentration curve for the urban public subsidy is almost diagonal (that is, benefits are neither pro-poor nor pro-rich), whereas the concentra-

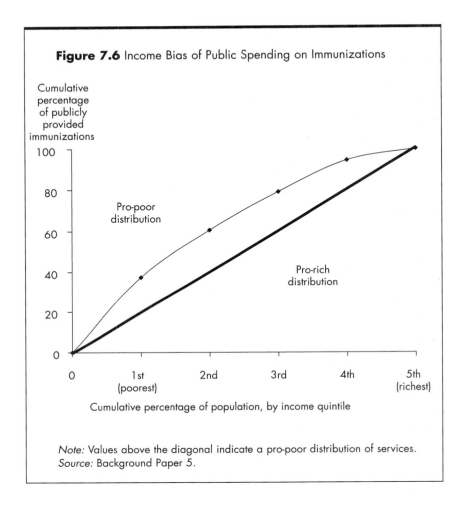

Figure 7.6 Income Bias of Public Spending on Immunizations

Cumulative percentage of publicly provided immunizations

Pro-poor distribution

Pro-rich distribution

Cumulative percentage of population, by income quintile

1st (poorest) 2nd 3rd 4th 5th (richest)

Note: Values above the diagonal indicate a pro-poor distribution of services.
Source: Background Paper 5.

tion curve for the rural population shows a pro-rich bias. Two features may explain this difference. Among the bottom income quintile, hospitalization rates (in both public and private facilities) are much higher in urban than in rural areas (1,266 versus 471 per 100,000). In the top income quintile, utilization rates are about the same (3,656 versus 3,269 per 100,000). Moreover, because private hospitals are more available in urban areas, the public sector utilization rate by the richest quintile is lower in urban than in rural areas.

These findings are consistent with those of other studies. A World Bank study (1997b) found that use of secondary care public hospitals, the most common type of hospital in rural areas, is low, largely because of poor quality and the lack of private sector alternatives. The study found that improving the quality of rural public hospitals would increase public sector utilization in rural areas.

Members of scheduled castes or scheduled tribes represent 29 percent of India's population and capture 28.4 percent of the subsidy benefits for curative care services. This suggests a fairly equal distribution of public services along caste and tribe affiliation lines.

State-Level Findings

Since curative care is primarily a state responsibility, one should expect health status outcomes and expenditure distributions to vary across states. Using the same National Sample Survey data, we repeated the utilization and benefit incidence analysis for 15 of the largest states and regions (which account for 97 percent of India's population); we based the analysis on income quintiles and poverty lines created for the urban and rural populations in each state (table 7.3). To simplify the presentation, we constructed a concentration index for each concentration curve to measure the level of inequality in subsidy benefits. The possible values of this index range from −1 (all benefits accrue to the poorest) to 1 (all benefits accrue to the richest); an index of 0 indicates that benefits are distributed evenly across income groups (Kakwani, Wagstaff, and van Doorslaer 1997).

In four states (Kerala, Gujarat, Tamil Nadu, and Maharashtra) curative care services are distributed nearly equally across income levels, with concentration indexes near zero. All other states reveal a pro-rich pattern of spending on curative care services, with Rs 2 or more going to the richest quintile for every Rs 1 that reaches the poorest quintile. In Bihar and Rajasthan Rs 5 or more of public health care spending is used by the top quintile for every Rs 1 that benefits the poorest quintile. The range of inequalities found in Indian states is similar to that found across developing countries (box 7.3).

Table 7.3 Income Bias in Public Spending on Curative Care in India and Selected States

STATE	CONCENTRATION INDEX[a]	SUBSIDY, RATIO OF RICHEST TO POOREST QUINTILE
Kerala	−0.041	1.10
Gujarat	0.001	1.14
Tamil Nadu	0.059	1.46
Maharashtra	0.060	1.21
Punjab	0.102	2.93
Andhra Pradesh	0.116	1.85
West Bengal	0.157	2.73
Haryana	0.201	2.98
Karnataka	0.208	3.58
National average	**0.214**	**3.28**
Northeast states	0.220	3.16
Orissa	0.282	4.87
Madhya Pradesh	0.292	4.16
Uttar Pradesh	0.304	4.09
Rajasthan	0.334	4.95
Bihar	0.419	10.30

Note: Northeast states consist of Assam, Arunachal Pradesh, Manipur, Meghalaya, Mizoram, Nagaland, and Tripura.
a. Possible values range from −1 (all benefits accrue to the poorest) to 1 (all benefits accrue to the richest); zero indicates equal distribution between income groups.
Source: Background Paper 18.

Box 7.3 Equity of Public Spending on Health: International Experience

International experience with measuring equity of public spending on health in developing countries indicates that:
- Public spending is most pro-poor at basic levels of social services.
- Discrimination by race, gender, caste, and minority status plays a role in utilization of publicly provided financed services.
- Some evidence supports the finding that public spending in the health sector appears to be more pro-poor in urban settings than in rural settings.

- Socialist countries have a better pro-poor record than nonsocialist countries.

These four findings are consistent with the new utilization and benefit incidence results from India.

The figure below compares the results of benefit incidence studies for India and for selected states in India with findings from other countries. Variations across countries in methodologies and sources of data make international comparisons difficult, but as the figure shows, the bulk of the findings point to public spending patterns in health that are not very pro-poor.

International Comparison of Inequalities in Health Sector Subsidies

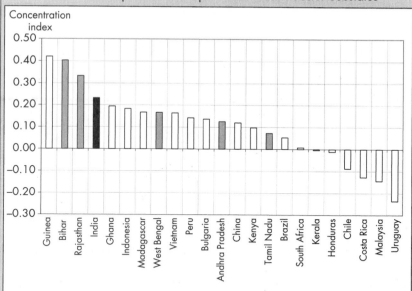

Note: Possible values range from −1 (all benefits accrue to the poorest) to 1 (all benefits accrue to the richest); zero indicates equal distribution between income groups. The shaded bars are values for India and selected states in India.

Inpatient care. Because inpatient care is the most costly health care service, analyzing state-level inpatient bed use by the poor provides the best way of comparing equity across states (box 7.4). In just two states, Maharashtra and Kerala, did the poor and the nonpoor spend about the same number of days in inpatient facilities. In all other states, people below the poverty accounted for a relatively small percentage of inpatient bed days, with the largest differences occurring in Bihar, Uttar Pradesh, Orissa, and the Northeastern states. These differences vary widely between urban and rural populations, with urban areas far more equitable than rural areas in all states.

Box 7.4 Adjusting Public Sector Hospitalization Rates for Income Bias, 1995–96

The number of public sector hospitalizations varies greatly across states in India, ranging from 2 per 1,000 in Bihar to 29 per 1,000 in Kerala. The pro-rich bias in hospitalization also varies across states, with Bihar having the most pro-rich distribution and Kerala being the only state to have a pro-poor distribution. Thus, some states that perform less well in terms of number of hospitalizations perform better when the number is adjusted to account for a pro-poor bias (an adjustment that produces a measure called "achievement"—see chapter 9, box 9.2). As shown in the figure below, Tamil Nadu, for example, has a lower public sector hospitalization rate than Orissa, but hospitalization in Tamil Nadu is much more concentrated among the poor. As a result, its achievement in public sector hospitalization is higher than Orissa's.

Of course, in many Indian states, a sizable proportion of hospitalizations are in the private sector. In Tamil Nadu, for example, only 40 percent of hospitalizations are in the public sector (in Orissa the proportion is nearly 90 percent). Taking into account the role of the private sector changes how states compare in terms of achievement. The achievement of Tamil Nadu's small but relatively equitable public sector is reinforced by a fairly large private sector, while the lack of achievement of Orissa's large but inequitable public sector is compounded by the fact that there is only a very small private sector.

Annual Hospitalization Rates and Achievement Indexes across Major Indian States

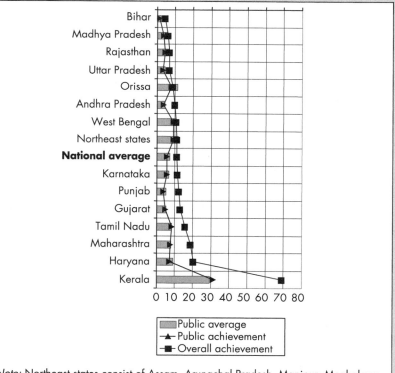

Note: Northeast states consist of Assam, Arunachal Pradesh, Manipur, Meghalaya, Mizoram, Nagaland, and Tripura.
Source: National Sample Survey Organisation (1998); authors' calculations.

Outpatient curative care. The National Sample Survey distinguishes between hospital-based outpatient care and care at primary health care facilities, but it does not disaggregate care provided by secondary and tertiary hospitals. On average, outpatient care is more equitable than inpatient care, but spending on hospital-based outpatient care is less equitably distributed than spending on outpatient care at primary care facilities (primary health centers, subcenters, and dispensaries).

The national average hides several important differences across states. In Rajasthan, Bihar, Haryana, and Madhya Pradesh, both hospital-based outpatient care and outpatient care at primary care facilities appear to favor people above the poverty line. These findings are consistent with anecdotal evidence that the poor join other groups in bypassing a failing primary care system. In West Bengal, Karnataka, Punjab, and the Northeastern states, hospital-based outpatient care favors people above the poverty line, while primary care favors people below the poverty line. The opposite is true in Andhra Pradesh and Gujarat, where hospital-based outpatient care favors people below the poverty line while primary care facilities favor those above the poverty line. Only in Maharashtra and Kerala do both types of outpatient care favor people below the poverty line.

This variability in the outpatient utilization data presents an important opportunity for policymakers to explore the determinants of equity performance. Important roles are perhaps being played by supply-side factors, such as placement of facilities, budget allocations, the level of facilities (secondary versus tertiary hospitals), and human resource and other input factors to improve quality. On the demand side, literacy and empowerment may influence poor households' likelihood of using public facilities.

Immunizations. The data reveal considerable variability across states in the use of preventive services such as immunization—a finding that is consistent with the National Family Health Surveys. Although public sector delivery of vaccines is pro-poor, not all of the poor are served: 37 percent of all unimmunized children are from the poorest income quintile, and Rajasthan, Bihar, and Uttar Pradesh have the highest proportions of children without immunizations. With the exception of Kerala and Tamil Nadu, which have few unimmunized children, and Uttar Pradesh, which has many, children below the poverty line are more likely not to be immunized than children above the poverty line.

Gender differences. Nationally, no clear bias against females is evident in public sector utilization. In fact, males account for 46.6 percent and females for 54.4 percent of total benefits from curative care services, even though males represent a higher percentage of the sample and curative care services included no pregnancy-related services. These national levels mask large variations across states, however, especially in rural areas. For example, in rural Gujarat, Punjab, and Haryana, men get more than 55 percent of the outpatient care, but in the Northeast states, they consume less than 45 percent.

How Does the Pattern of Public Spending Affect Health Outcomes?

Without some form of public action, the poor will be left without critical health services. Relying on private provision alone will not be equitable—it will not provide all Indians with a basic standard of health care nor will it allocate health care spending proportionally to all income groups. While some states have ensured that public financing is not skewed to the rich, many more states are doing too little to ensure that the poor have access to and use health services. In these states, overall public financing of health services is not equitable, and the public health system tends to respond more to the demands of richer Indians than to the poor.

Alongside the question of whether the distribution of health services and health financing is fair is the question of whether fairness in public financing of health makes a difference in other health outcomes. We examined the relationship of state-level rates of infant and child mortality to the concentration index derived from public hospitalization. After adjustment for other factors influencing mortality—state per capita income, literacy levels, and per capita public spending on health—the analysis showed that a pro-poor distribution is significantly associated with reduced infant and child mortality (see appendix table 7A.1). The analysis also suggests that the distribution of public resources may be more important in influencing mortality than the amounts of public health spending, at least over the range of public health spending provided by states in 1995–96 (amounts ranging from Rs 57 per capita in Bihar to Rs 132 in Kerala). Although we don't fully understand the mechanisms that explain the relationship between more equitable public health services and better health outcomes, the results highlight the importance of equity in improving health outcomes and the need to further study and monitor equity and health system outcomes.

Appendix

Table 7A.1 Infant and Child Mortality among Indian States: Effects of Public Hospitalization, Equity, and Other Factors, 1995–96

INDICATOR	INFANT MORTALITY		CHILD MORTALITY	
	COEFFICIENT (STANDARD ERROR)	t STATISTIC (p VALUE)	COEFFICIENT (STANDARD ERROR)	t STATISTIC (p VALUE)
Intercept	88.26	n.a.	24.47	n.a.
State public hospitals	92.08	2.19	44.48	3.20
Concentration index	(42.04)	(.05)	(13.91)	(.008)
State per capita income (rupees)	−0.001	−.36	−0.0009	−.79
	(.003)	(.72)	(.001)	(.40)
State per capita public health spending (rupees)	−0.10	−.89	−2.97	−.17
	(.12)	(.39)	(17.63)	(.90)
State literacy rate (percent)	−43.32	−.81	−0.08	−2.01
	(53.3)	(.43)	(.039)	(.07)
R-squared	.75		.83	

n.a. Not applicable.
Note: Infant mortality is for those up to one year of age; child mortality is for those age one year to just under age five.

Notes

1. These data do not imply that the programs could prevent the same proportion of deaths and DALYs (disability-adjusted life years) lost. We count only the direct deaths and disability related to these conditions and do not estimate their effects as risk factors for other diseases. For example, vitamin A deficiency and protein energy malnutrition contribute to a larger loss of life than is directly attributed to them because they also contribute to pneumonia, diarrhea, and measles.

2. An effective tobacco control program also involves taxing tobacco products, restricting advertising, and providing smoking cessation interventions. Dietary advice and exercise promotion are also low-cost interventions that are part of related programs aimed at reducing cardiovascular disease. The prevention of injury involves public education; engineering solutions, such as improving road safety; and regulatory measures, such as requiring the installation and use of seatbelts and enforcing speed limits and drunk driving laws. Fire-related injuries and deaths are concentrated among women of reproductive age; this condition reflects their exposure to domestic violence, as well as to kitchen fires, and requires interventions tailored to address violence against women in traditional and modern settings.

3. Since the Fifth Five-Year Plan, national resources have been used to supplement rural health infrastructure (particularly for sub-centers, primary health centers, and community health centers); some urban clinics; and rural health personnel (particularly auxiliary nurse midwives). Successive World Bank–supported India Population Projects have facilitated this process, as states received 90 percent of these credits. In part, these investments were intended to support centrally sponsored programs and provide the first level of curative care more generally.

4. The benefit incidence is calculated in the following manner. First, rank all individuals (or households) from poorest to richest by the chosen measure of current welfare. Then identify which individuals use each type of publicly provided service and calculate the average unit cost of providing each type of service (net of cost recovery fees). Then multiply the utilization figures by the government's unit cost of provision (net of fees) to derive the amount of public spending on the good or service going to each group. Mathematically:

$$X_j \equiv \sum_i U_{ij} \frac{S_i}{U_i} \equiv \frac{U_{ij}}{U_i} S_i \equiv \sum_i e_{ij} S_i$$

X_j = health sector subsidy enjoyed by group j
U_{ij} = utilization of service i by group j
U_i = utilization of service i by all groups combined
S_i = government net expenditure on service i
e_{ij} = group j's share of utilization of service i

5. The share of the population reported here as living below the poverty line is based on the 16 largest states and regions. The 34 percent figure reported in chapter 4 is based on the entire population.

6. The analysis measures costs per type of visit using standardized unit-cost data rather than actual expenditures. That is, if a primary health center had only one patient per year, the analysis would not attribute all the cost of inpatient beds to that one patient. Using budget data to distribute expenditures to different levels of facilities produces similar results (Background Paper 5).

CHAPTER 8

Financing Health

In this chapter we address three financing mechanisms: revenue raising, resource intermediation (including pooling), and resource allocation and purchasing.[1] As a prelude, we give a detailed picture of the amount and sources of financing for private and public elements of the health sector and the unique structure of financing responsibilities in the public sector. As in the other chapters, the dominant questions are: How much are the poor protected? And what are the appropriate roles for the public and private sectors? See box 8.1 for a summary of the empirical findings and policy challenges discussed in the chapter.

Health Sector Spending

In 1996, India spent about 4.5 percent of its GDP on health, less than the average of 5.6 percent for low- and middle-income countries.[2] India also has one of the highest proportions of private health financing anywhere in the world, about 82 percent. Only five countries (Cambodia, the Democratic Republic of the Congo, Georgia, Myanmar, and Sierra Leone) have a higher dependence on private financing in the health sector (WHO 2000c). The low spending (about $18 per capita) and the dominance of private sources of financing make India unique (World Bank 1997b; WHO 2000c).

Box 8.1 Empirical Findings and Policy Challenges

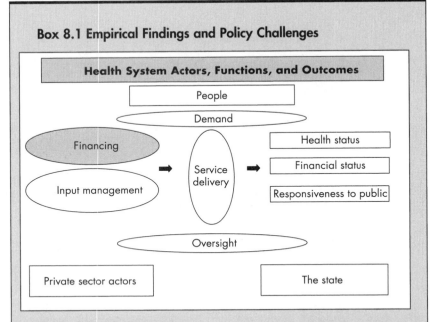

Empirical Findings

- Overall health spending in India is estimated at 4.5 percent of GDP, less than the average of 5.6 percent for low- and middle-income countries.
- Public spending on health in India is 0.9 percent of GDP, among the lowest in the world .
- Out-of-pocket private spending dominates health expenditures, with 82 percent of all health spending from private sources.
- Hospitalization frequently results in financial catastrophe, especially in the absence of risk pooling. About 10 percent of Indians, most of them employees in government or elsewhere in the formal sector, have some form of health insurance.
- The gap in public financing for health between rich and poor states is widening and threatening to expand the gaps in outcomes.

> **Policy Challenges**
> - How will India expand public spending on basic health services to improve quality of services and the health of the poor?
> - How can regional inequalities in health sector spending be decreased given decentralized financing and differences in implementation capacities?
> - How will India be able to shift from predominantly private out-of-pocket health financing to risk-pooling mechanisms, particularly when incomes are low and most people belong to rural informal sectors?
> - How can India develop the regulatory environment and information systems to oversee new health financing mechanisms?

India's public expenditures on health are even further below international levels than its overall spending— 0.9 percent of GDP, compared with an average of 2.8 percent for low- and middle-income countries and a global average of 5.5 percent (World Bank 1997b).[3] The government's fiscal effort, measured as the proportion of total government expenditure spent on health, again identifies India as a low performer—13th from the bottom when compared with all other countries (WHO 2000c).

Over the 1985–2000 period, India's public spending on health rose in inflation-adjusted per capita terms, but it fell as a share of GDP (figure 8.1). Even if the share of GDP had remained at 1.1 percent, the level at the start of the period, it would still rank among the lowest in the world.

Given India's size and decentralized political structure, patterns of public spending on health must be examined at the state level. In fact, the financing responsibility for public spending is primarily at the state level with some overlapping responsibilities with the central government on a series of centrally sponsored schemes (chapter

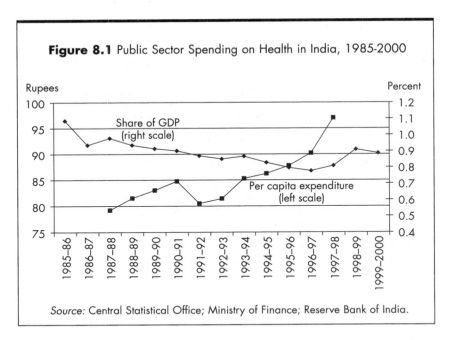

Figure 8.1 Public Sector Spending on Health in India, 1985-2000

Source: Central Statistical Office; Ministry of Finance; Reserve Bank of India.

7). Several facts are evident from the distribution of public spending by state and source (figure 8.2):

- States vary widely in overall per capita public spending on health— in Kerala and Punjab, for example, spending is double that in Bihar, Madhya Pradesh, and Uttar Pradesh.

- Public spending per capita is lowest in the poorest states (Bihar, Madhya Pradesh, and Uttar Pradesh).

- States typically account for about 75 percent of total public spending per capita for health and thus are the major determinants of the variation in such spending.

- The central government's share of health spending is considerably more equally distributed than is the state share, but is slightly tilted away from the poorer states.[4]

Although data on per capita spending by state do not address the important dimension of how resources are spent, the size of the dif-

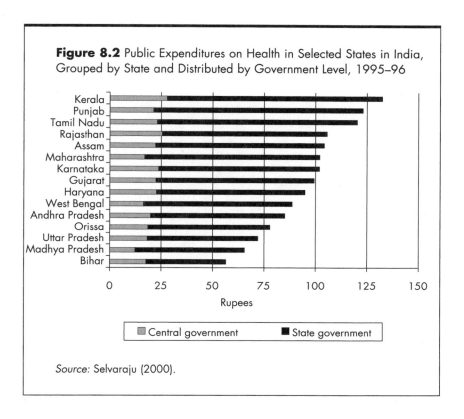

Figure 8.2 Public Expenditures on Health in Selected States in India, Grouped by State and Distributed by Government Level, 1995–96

Source: Selvaraju (2000).

ferences and the pro-rich distributions have serious long-term implications. With health financing a major responsibility of state governments, spending per capita will inevitably be lower in the poorer states than elsewhere. The challenge for the national government is to consider a variety of policy instruments, including centrally sponsored schemes, equalization funds, and other fiscal incentives to address the inequalities perpetuated by the current financing arrangements.

State variations in private spending on health services (figure 8.3) are equally impressive:

• In Kerala and Punjab, per capita private spending is almost four times larger than in Rajasthan and Bihar.

- While there is some consistency between the high a low level of private and public spending (Bihar and Orissa low, and Kerala and Punjab high), some states have different rankings between the two.

- Private facilities receive the lion share of out-of-pocket expenditures.

Here again, the amount of money paid for health services does not capture individuals' choices of type of provider or quality of care purchased (both issues addressed in chapters 6 and 7). Policymakers should, however, be concerned with the large state-level variations,

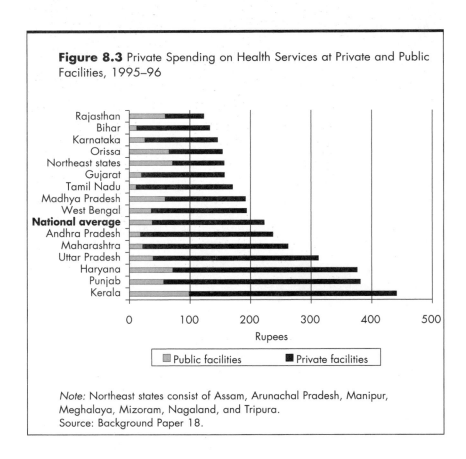

Figure 8.3 Private Spending on Health Services at Private and Public Facilities, 1995–96

Note: Northeast states consist of Assam, Arunachal Pradesh, Manipur, Meghalaya, Mizoram, Nagaland, and Tripura.
Source: Background Paper 18.

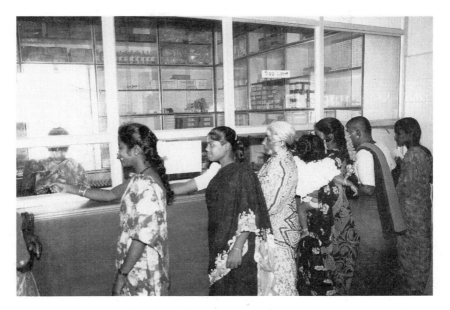

Lining up to receive drugs at a dispensary (PHOTOGRAPH BY GEETANJALI CHOPRA/ HEMANT MEHTA/THE WORLD BANK)

which may lead to increasing the gaps in outcomes for the three types of health system objectives (improved health status, financial protection, and consumer satisfaction), addressed in the next chapter. The determinants of private spending include the relationship between income and demand for services, the impact of education on health-seeking behavior, the availability of alternative providers, and the quality (actual or perceived) of both private and public sector providers.

One determinant of high private spending on health in India is low public spending on health. The state-level relationship between public and private spending appears, however, to be more complex (figure 8.4). In Bihar and Orissa, both public and private spending on health appear to be relatively low, while in Kerala, Punjab, and Maharashtra, spending is relatively high for both. The size of spending appears to move in different directions for Rajasthan and Tamil Nadu (high public, low private) and for Uttar Pradesh and Andhra Pradesh (high private, low public).

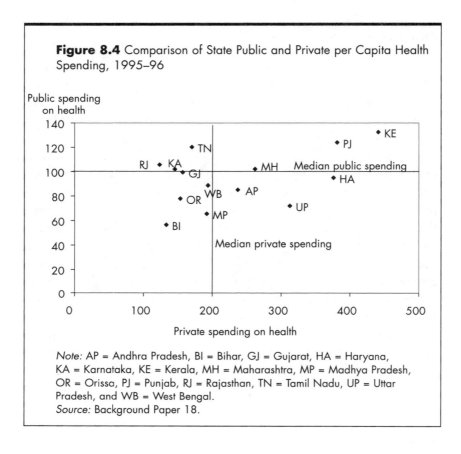

Figure 8.4 Comparison of State Public and Private per Capita Health Spending, 1995–96

Note: AP = Andhra Pradesh, BI = Bihar, GJ = Gujarat, HA = Haryana, KA = Karnataka, KE = Kerala, MH = Maharashtra, MP = Madhya Pradesh, OR = Orissa, PJ = Punjab, RJ = Rajasthan, TN = Tamil Nadu, UP = Uttar Pradesh, and WB = West Bengal.
Source: Background Paper 18.

Financing Mechanisms

One way of thinking about the basic functions of financing the health sector is to segregate them into three categories:

- Mechanisms for raising resources for the sector.

- Mechanisms for organizing clusters of funds as resources flow from sources to providers of care.

- Mechanisms for resource allocation that influences which providers receive the relative shares of available funds.

Structure of the Flow of Funds

A useful first step in analyzing the different financing mechanisms is to understand the architecture of the health care financing system. Several state-level health account activities provide a strong foundation for exploring the structure of financial flows (Background Paper 1; Sharma, McGreevey, and Hotchkiss 2000).

In Rajasthan (appendix figure 8A.1), about 71 percent of total health spending is from private sources, a level smaller than the national average but one that still dominates Rajasthan's spending picture. Another critical feature is the shared responsibility between the central government and the state governments. Detailed analysis found that over the past two decades about 73 percent of total public resources for health have been provided directly by state governments (World Bank 1997b). Recent estimates show the share of states may have increased to account for 75–78 percent of total public sector health spending.

For private financing, the out-of-pocket share of the flow of funds dominates and for the most part is not pooled through insurance mechanisms. Here again, this dominant form of financing has strong negative implications for equity and increases the risk that vulnerable groups will slip into poverty.

Revenue Generation

As is the case in other low-income countries, the government in India has an intractable problem in mobilizing adequate resources when much of the population is poor. Taxation and the pooling of funds for health insurance is made difficult by the low rate of participation in the formal labor market and the large, informal rural labor market. Cost recovery accounts for a very small share of public sector expenditure; the bulk of resources come from general revenues.[5] Only three states—Kerala, Punjab, and Haryana—have cost recovery ratios close to 10 percent, while for all other states the ratio is less than 4 percent (appendix table 8A.1). The bulk of the fees for public facility care (more than 80 percent) were paid by the richest

40 percent of the population. The progressive cost recovery system was consistent for both urban and rural populations. That the rich pay more may reflect the fact that the rich use services more (chapter 7) or that the quality of care provided to those who pay may be higher than for those who do not pay.

Assessments of the cost recovery system in several states have uncovered weaknesses (World Bank 1997b):

- The states have no appropriate institutional framework for reviewing user charges.

- The level of cost recovery is minimal because of low fees and inadequate collection mechanisms.

- Mechanisms for exempting the poor from user charges are difficult to target and implement.

- No adequate mechanisms exist to ensure that recovered funds would be used at the point of collection—and thus serve as an incentive to operate efficiently—rather than being sent to the government treasury.

Those in the richest 20 percent of the population spent, on average, five times more than did those in the poorest 20 percent (appendix figure 8A.2). Similarly, those above the poverty line spent three times more than did those below it (appendix figure 8A.3). Individuals not belonging to a scheduled caste or tribe spent, on average, Rs 100 more than others. Urban residents spent Rs 100 more than rural residents.

An important consequence of these differences in out-of-pocket health spending is that when combined with the low use of "free" public services by the most vulnerable groups, the access to health care services appears to be severely limited. A second concern is the hardship created by the mode of resource generation by the private sector (fee for service paid directly by the patient) and the limited availability of resource pooling; this is discussed in more detail in the next section. Out-of-pocket spending depletes savings and assets and forces borrowing to cover medical bills, especially inpatient bills.

Intermediation and Pooling Mechanisms

One argument for pooling resources in the health sector is that it spreads risks across insured populations— an important consideration in India because of the current huge financial risks involved with hospitalization (box 8.2). In one year, about one-quarter of all hospitalized Indians may fall into poverty because of the costs of medical care (chapter 9). Pooling becomes increasingly important as the epidemiological transition takes place in India and health services provision changes from low cost per episode to high cost per episode. As was shown in chapter 3 (box 3.4), many countries are taking steps to pool risks and subsidize health care for the sick and the poor.

Box 8.2 How Hospitalization Can Devastate

Krishna is 30 years old and lives in Katkol, a rural village in Karnataka. Six months ago Krishna fell while harvesting coconuts at a plantation. He lost consciousness, and his left leg started to bleed. The plantation owner immediately took Krishna to the primary health center, where the Medical Officer gave him first aid and asked them to go to the city of Mysore because the nearby hospital did not have facilities to attend to him.

Krishna's employer took him to Mysore in his car; with the Medical Officer's referral letter, Krishna was immediately admitted into the government hospital. He was given saline solution and after two days regained full consciousness. Krishna was told that his back had been injured and that he would receive surgery the next day.

Box 8.2 (continued)

After the operation, Krishna stayed in the hospital for almost four months. During that time his wounds became worse, his legs swelled, and big bedsores formed on his back, which was full of pus. The hospital provided some medicines, but he was also asked to purchase more injections and glucose "bottles."

Krishna described his hospital experience as being very unpleasant. Basic amenities like drinking water were not available. Paramedics and other staff were hostile and would shout because Krishna's family could not give money when they demanded it. His elder brother and his wife came to look after him and had to sleep on the floor and eat in a hotel. The doctors would come to see him once every two days.

Eventually he was told that he would not live for more than two months and that the hospital could not do anything more for him. He was asked to leave because of a shortage of beds, and the family hired a car to take Krishna home.

For Krishna's hospitalization, the family incurred expenses of Rs 15,000—on transportation, medicines, food, and tips to health staff and doctors. The family has an annual income of about Rs 6,000. The funds for hospitalization were raised by selling the half-acre of land they had and also by taking a loan at the rate of 10 percent per month.

Krishna now sleeps with his back facing up, and all his wounds on his back and legs are oozing. He has become pale and weak, and the family expects him to die at any moment.

Source: Administrative Staff College of India (1995).

Insurance mechanisms, however, are not without risks of market failure (Background Paper 2). Several characteristics of the health care market may lead to cost escalation:

- Information gaps between providers and patients may create incentives to provide more care than may be medically appropriate, especially in a regime of pure indemnity insurance. The information gaps make the patient, and insurers for that matter, less willing to question the doctor's recommendations (Arrow 1963). The problem will be greater in situations in which the patient can choose his or her doctor and treatment freely and then present the bill to the insurer for reimbursement.

- Health insurance reduces the incentive of individuals to guard against poor health and thus tends to drive up demand for more expensive care. The covered individual may know that he or she is taking more risks, but the insurance company may not (the insurance term used for this information gap is "moral hazard").

- Another information gap is that patients are likely to know much more about their health status and future needs than insurers. Thus, people expecting to incur significant health expenditures in the near future will figure disproportionately among those who choose to get insured (the insurance term used for this information gap factor is "adverse selection").

- Without minimum capital reserves and incomplete epidemiological information about the population, which is the case in most developing countries, insurance companies risk long-term failure by guessing wrong and charging premiums that are too low in comparison to the benefits offered in a competitive environment.

- Empirical evidence exists that health spending per capita is positively associated with the proportion of the population covered by private insurance.

The contribution of an insurance scheme, whether public or private, to improving the quality of health care depends on whether the scheme is able to influence the licensing of medical personnel and facilities and the entry of highly skilled individuals into the health sector. For equity, the main concern is that private insurers will try to sell only to low-risk customers. But an expansion of private health insurance could eventually improve access to public facilities by those unable to get private insurance.

The insurance schemes in India can be sorted into four broad groups: mandatory, voluntary, employer-based, and NGO-based (Garg 2001). The four types of scheme together cover roughly about 10 percent of India's population (appendix table 8A.2).

Mandatory health insurance schemes. The mandatory schemes consist of the Employees State Insurance Scheme (ESIS), for certain low-income employees of the organized industrial sector, and the Central Government Health Scheme (CGHS), mainly for central government employees. Both these schemes are principally financed by the contributions of beneficiaries and their employers and from taxes. The ESIS receives some contribution from state governments, whereas the CGHS is mainly financed from central government revenues. ESIS covered 35.4 million beneficiaries in 1998 and CGHS covered 4.4 million beneficiaries in 1996. Providers are mainly salaried, and hospitals work under global budgets.

Voluntary health insurance schemes. Voluntary schemes are for individuals and corporations, and are available mainly through the General Insurance Corporation (GIC) of India—a government-owned monopoly—and its four subsidiaries. These schemes are financed from household and corporate funds. GIC offers one policy for groups and mostly nonpoor individuals and another mostly for poor individuals and families. These policies have had only limited success in India; in 1996 they covered only 1.7 million people. With the passage of the Insurance Regulatory and Development Authority Act of 1999 and the liberalization of insurance, more private voluntary health schemes are expected to be available in the near future.

Employer-based schemes. Public and private sector companies offer health insurance through their own employer-managed facilities by way of lump sum payments, reimbursement of employees' health expenditures, or coverage under one of the GIC policies. Workers buy health insurance through their employers. Ellis, Alam, and Gupta (2000) estimate that roughly 30 million people are covered under employer-based schemes.

Community-based insurance schemes. Primarily for the informal sector, community-based schemes tend to offer coverage for all available services but emphasize primary health care (box 8.3). Most of these schemes are financed from patient collections, government grants, donations, and miscellaneous items such as interest earnings or employment schemes. Most NGOs have their own facilities or mobile clinics to provide health care. Total coverage is estimated to be about 30 million people (Ellis, Alam, and Gupta 2000).

Table 8.1 summarizes the main market failures in the financing of health care, the consequences, and the policy measures for correcting them.

Box 8.3 Innovative Health Insurance Schemes in India

Up to 10 percent of the people in India, most of them in government and other industries in the formal sector, are covered by some form of health insurance, but the policy benefits are limited and claims service is poor. A few innovative schemes have been tried out across the country to address the needs of the larger segment of self-employed and informal workers. Among them are the following plans:

- *Ambikpur Health Association,* Orissa: Free outpatient care and limited hospitalization are provided to about 75,000 individuals on a voluntary basis. Among the innovative features of the plan are screening at the time of enrolment to avoid adverse selection of participants. However,

Box 8.3 (continued)

premiums cover only 1-2 percent of the plan's outreach costs.

- *Mallur Milk Co-operative*, Karnataka: Covering a population of 7,000 spread across three villages, the scheme provides preventive and curative health care (both outpatient and inpatient) to all eligible community members. Participation is mandatory. Income from an endowment fund covers all expenses.
- *Sewagram*, Maharashtra: Free primary care, drugs, referrals, and hospitalization for nonchronic conditions are provided to a population of more than 14,000 spread across 12 villages (75 percent mandatory attendance within a participating village). Sliding-scale premiums are employed to promote equity.
- *Meloj Milk Co-operative*, Gujarat: Outpatient consultation, discounted drugs, and diagnostic services are provided by Aga Khan Health Services. Enrollment is mandatory for all co-op members.

Among the complex issues and problems these organizations face, two are of particular importance: (a) arranging for cost-recovery without excluding the poor and (b) dealing with moral hazard and adverse selection. These issues have been addressed by these organizations with varying degrees of success. In addition to the protection from financial shock that they provide to their members, these plans have sometimes also helped to enhance the allocative efficiency of health spending by developing low-cost treatments or by increasing the utilization of preventive care.

Source: Ranson (1999).

Table 8.1 Market Failures, Consequences, and Responses in Financing Health Care

MARKET FAILURE	CONSEQUENCES	MEASURES TO CORRECT FAILURE
Demand side		
Moral hazard	Overuse of services by patients	Deductible, co-insurance, co-payments, etc.; gatekeepers, waiting lines
Adverse selection	Little risk pooling. No insurance market will exist; only some insured	Tax subsidy, compulsory universal coverage. Lifetime enrollment
Underuse of health care	Underuse of services with lumpy costs by poor and also underuse of preventive care and of care for diseases with externalities	Education, information, and communication; free or subsidized care
Supply side		
Supplier-induced demand	Increased demand by patients; raises costs of care	Use provider payment mechanisms such as salaries, global budgets, and case payments
Risk selection (skimming)	No insurance for disabled, sick, poor, and elderly	Open enrollment, community ratings, risk-adjusted premiums for individuals, compulsory or social insurance
Skimping	Deny benefits to the sick	Social insurance, redress procedures
Exclusions	Exclude pre-existing conditions and certain diseases for stipulated period or life of the contract	Lifetime and compulsory insurance, guaranteed renewability
Monopoly or insurance cartel	Excess profit, poor quality products, underproduction	Antitrust laws

Linking health insurance to employment in an organization will not provide extensive coverage in India because most people are self-employed, or do not have a formal employer or steady employment. Many of the poor are excluded from access to high quality health care and health insurance because of inability to pay, lack of knowledge, or other factors related to geography or discrimination. Growing international experience with insuring the informal sector shows some possibilities and limitations that can complement India's own experience (box 8.4).

Box 8.4 International Experience with Health Insurance for the Informal Sector

Providing health care and financial protection for people who do not work in the formal sector—those who do not have regular salaried jobs with social security or employment benefits and taxed incomes—are major challenges in most low-income countries. In surveys worldwide, workers in the informal sector regularly single out health insurance as their greatest insurance need. Experiments in China and Tanzania are two examples of how countries have dealt with this challenge:

In China, rural health insurance covers hospital and primary health care costs through private and public contributions. Premiums paid by beneficiaries are supplemented through a village public welfare fund and government subsidies.

In Tanzania, a pilot project provides health insurance through five mutual associations of workers in the informal sector. A key feature of successful contributory insurance schemes for the informal sector is their organization around an association based on trust and mutual support (professional group, village) and the administrative capacity to collect contributions and provide benefits.

Some of the lessons learned from health insurance schemes in the informal sector:

- Risk pools that cover only a few communities or only the poor often do not have sufficient economies of scale to be financially viable and are not able to provide cross-subsidies and withstand high demands for catastrophic care.
- The success of a risk pooling scheme is dependant on the quality and range of health services provided and the degree of accountability to the community.
- The collection and management of revenues is often inefficient and thereby reduces the funds available for investment or for providing services.
- Exclusion from an insurance scheme can be a big problem; preventing unreasonable exclusion requires the capacity to regulate (for example, making participation mandatory, making contributions non-risk-related) or to provide financial incentives (for example, provide subsidies for the poor to join).

Source: World Bank (2000e); WHO (2000c).

As the health sector in India reacts to liberalization in the insurance market, the policy challenges are immense. The large and predominantly fee-for-services nature of private sector spending will continue to dominate in the short and medium term. But the transformation into more pooling is inevitable; it will bring with it the potential for improvements in efficiency and equity in the health sector as well as risks of escalating costs and of widening the gap between rich and poor. Essential tasks for policymakers to meet these challenges include laying the groundwork for appropriate policy measures and building the institutional capacity to implement them.

Box 8.5 Conclusions of the National Seminar on Health Insurance

In anticipation of the passage of the Insurance Regulatory and Development Authority Act of 1999, the government of India held a seminar for senior policymakers on health insurance. The objectives of the seminar, which was held on November 16–17, 1999, were to understand the potential risks and benefits of private health insurance and to identify what the government should do to ensure that social objectives are met with the liberalization of health insurance.

The approach proposed by the seminar was to support voluntary insurance rather than expand existing social insurance schemes. The likely impact on the poor was not clear. They could benefit from an expansion of quality in the private sector, or the gap in access to quality care might increase; the risk also remains of subsidizing the wealthy.

Pro-Poor Recommendations
- Reduce the public subsidy to the wealthy by charging the full cost of service to the insured who use private insurance, finance the regulatory agency through premiums, and reduce or eliminate tax incentives for private insurance, particularly indemnity based insurance.
- Define a minimum package of covered services that includes preventive, maternity, and catastrophic cases in order to prevent such cases from being relegated to the public sector.
- Encourage informal community financing schemes that have less regulation and lower capital deposit requirements (such as managed care schemes through NGOs) and assess other financing options for the poor.

Health Systems Recommendations
- Establish a specialized regulatory agency for health insurance that would define benefits packages, ensure the transparency and comparability of packages, define treatment protocols, ensure guaranteed renewal of policies, reduce ability to deny coverage on the basis of pre-existing conditions, establish conflict resolution mechanisms, promote community financing, and monitor the performance of different schemes.
- Develop quality assurance procedures in health care.

Resources and Allocation and Purchasing Mechanisms

The third set of financing mechanisms relates to resource decisions in the public and private health sectors. Recent work on resource allocation and purchasing has identified a number of questions that can help public sector policymakers fine-tune their decisions and improve the oversight of both the private and public sector (Preker, Harding, and Travis 2000). The questions include what the resources are being spent on and for whom; the nature of the allocation and purchasing mechanisms; and institutional arrangements governing resource allocation and purchasing transactions (appendix table 8A.3).

The health sector in a number of states, as well as through centrally sponsored schemes, has experimented with different forms of contracting with the private sector (for-profit and not-for-profit providers). These forms ranged from contracting for nonmedical services (box 8.6) to purchasing medical services such as cataract surgeries and leprosy rehabilitation. Other examples have included the purchase of laboratory services and media and sensitization campaigns. Policy research should pay attention not only to the efficiencies of various purchasing and contracting arrangements but also to the institutional requirements for their success.

Box 8.6 Contracting Out Nonclinical Hospital Services to the Private Sector: Experiences from Karnataka

The Karnataka Department of Health has been contracting out a set of nonclinical services for 82 secondary level hospitals in hopes of improving the maintenance of their facilities in a cost-effective way. The pilot initiative began in 1997 and is part of the Karnataka Health Systems Development Project, which is supported by the World Bank.

The services contracted include building cleaning and maintenance and waste management. The contracts were let in a competitive bidding process, and monthly payments to the vendors are based on satisfactory performance. The experience has been generally encouraging to the Department of Health. The government is no longer recruiting unskilled labor for the tasks being contracted out, and it plans to expand the scheme. Displaced staff members have been transferred or retrained as ambulance or operating theater assistants. Overall, the contract payments have been less than the salaries they replaced.

Some findings from a recent evaluation of the pilot scheme:

- Patients and hospital staff reported that the level of cleanliness in the hospitals had improved and recommended continuation of the pilot scheme.
- Performance was most satisfactory for lower-skilled and visible tasks such as maintenance of corridors, wards, and toilets and for those that required less financial input, such as minor repairs, replacements, and maintenance of exteriors.
- Performance was less satisfactory in areas requiring technical competence or larger financial inputs or both, such as waste management, providing supplies, maintaining safety (repairing leaks), and displaying information.

One of the main recommendations was that better performance and compliance is contingent on strengthening the capacity of hospital staff to supervise the work and training those working in more complex areas of waste management.

Experience from several countries indicates that the early phases of contracting often involve problems of adjustment and that benefits tend to go up over time as the managers of contracts get more experience.

Another consistent finding is that the price of the contract needs to be sufficient to provide adequate service. If the price is too low, then the service will never be adequate, whether it is provided in-house or contracted out. Under some of the catering contracts at hospitals in other state health system development projects in India, food quality and quantity reportedly declined after being contracted out because the services were priced too low.

Conclusions

While the consultative process that launched the studies for this report focused attention in the area of health finance on the challenges of insurance, the data presented here have raised other challenges. By international standards, India's commitment to public financing of critical health and public health services appears to be very low (0.9 percent of GDP for all public spending on health). The weakness of public funding may have contributed to the dominance of private financing, which overwhelmingly is out-of-pocket fee-for-service payments by patients; such payments put the poor at higher financial risk and skew the provision of critical health services to the richest. The inequities and distortions will become more apparent in chapter 9, where we pursue the issues of financial risks and fairness in health in greater detail.

Another striking finding relates to the astonishing variations across states in both public and private spending, with some states spending up to four times more per capita than others. A critical challenge for India is to find ways to improve the distribution of resources, especially for priority public health activities and services, to ensure that poorer states do not lag behind as much in terms of resources and capacity.

The state-level analysis in this chapter is but one dimension of a needed countrywide public expenditure review in the health sector. Given the large variations in state-level commitments to public spending, differences are to be expected in how the resources are spent. But as shown in this report, the challenge facing India is not only a question of increasing public spending on health but of finding the mechanisms to raise resources, pool risks, and purchase care that will protect the poor and the sick and be more efficient in driving the health system in the future.

Appendix

Table 8A.1 Health Expenditures and Cost Recovery in the Public Sector of Selected States, 1996

(100,000 rupees except as noted)

STATE	TOTAL EXPENDITURES	TOTAL USER FEES	PERCENTAGE OF COSTS RECOVERED
Andhra Pradesh	47,898	735	1.53
Bihar	22,130	230	1.03
Gujarat	33,564	438	1.31
Haryana	11,957	1,137	9.51
Himachal Pradesh	11,621	784	0.67
Karnataka	42,614	1,180	2.77
Kerala	31,226	4,952	15.86
Madhya Pradesh	36,218	578	1.60
Maharashtra	45,893	2,127	4.63
Northeast states	22,695	386	1.70
Orissa	19,093	183	0.96
Punjab	17,693	1,888	10.67
Rajasthan	43,161	398	0.92
Tamil Nadu	55,984	1,238	2.21
Uttar Pradesh	84,308	2,726	3.23
West Bengal	50,802	1,063	2.09

Note: Northeast states consist of Assam, Arunachal Pradesh, Manipur, Meghalaya, Mizoram, Nagaland, and Tripura.
Source: Background Paper 5.

Table 8A.2 Salient Features of Some Insurance Schemes in India

	MANDATORY SOCIAL INSURANCE SCHEMES		VOLUNTARY PRIVATE INSURANCE—MEDICLAIM	EMPLOYER-BASED SCHEME	COMMUNITY-BASED INSURANCE/NGOS
INDICATORS	ESIS	CGHS			
Beneficiaries	Factory sector employees with income of less than Rs 6,500 per month (their dependants are also covered)	Employees of central government—current and retired, some autonomous and quasigovernmental organizations, MPs, judges, freedom fighters, journalists	• Individuals and groups with persons ages 5 to 75 years. • Children between 3 months and 5 years covered with parents.	Public and private sector employees	People in the communities
Coverage	About 35.3 million beneficiaries in 1998	About 4.4 million beneficiaries in 1996	• 1.7 million beneficiaries • Urban poor and groups more likely to purchase policy	About 30 million beneficiaries in 1999	• About 30 million beneficiaries in 1999 • Normally quarter of eligible populations targeted
Benefits	• Medical benefits, cash benefits. • Preventive and promotive care, and health education.	• All outpatient facilities, preventive and promotive care available in dispensaries • Inpatient facilities available in government hospitals and in approved private hospitals on being referred	• Hospitalization according to benefit level • Exclusions and waiting period • Maternity benefits allowed with extra premium	Categorized under • GHIP • Reimbursements • Lump-sum payments • Own facilities	Mainly preventive care; also ambulatory and inpatient care.

Premiums (financing of scheme)	• 4.75 % of employee wages paid by employers • 1.75 % of employee wages paid by employees • 12.5 % of total expenses paid by state governments	• Vary from Rs 15 to Rs 150 per month according to salary • Mainly financed by central government	Premiums based on age and benefit level		• Financed by patient collection, government grants, and donations • Premiums depend on the scheme—flat rate or income-based
Provider payments	• Mainly salaries for physicians in dispensaries and referral hospitals • Hospitals have global budget financed by ESIS through state governments.	• Salaries for doctors • Providers not allowed private practice • Treatment in private hospitals is reimbursed on case basis subject to actual expenditure and prescribed ceilings.	Indemnity type—insured pays to the provider who is later reimbursed according to the benefit level.	Based on benefits	Mainly fee for service
				• Salaries to providers in own facilities • Fee for service by patients, covered partly or wholly by the company	
Administrative costs	About 21% of revenue expenditure for employee wages, administering cash benefits, revenue recovery, and implementation in new area	• Direct administrative costs including travel expenditure, office expenses— 5% of total expenditure • Part of salaries can also be charged to administrative costs.	• Generally high • Low claim-premium ratio because a large proportion of funds are spent on administration or kept as profits	Depends on the scheme implemented by the company (will be highest for own facilities)	Generally low (3–5% depending on the scheme)

Note: ESIS, Employees State Insurance Scheme; CGHS, Central Government Health Scheme; NGOs, nongovernmental organizations; GHIP, Group Health Insurance Program.
Source: Background Paper 1.

Table 8A.3 Questions for Policymakers to Ask when Deciding on Resource Allocations and Purchasing

ISSUE	QUESTIONS
Core policy characteristics	• Demand (for whom to buy?) • Supply (what to buy, in what form, and what to exclude?) • Prices and incentive regime (at what price and how to pay?)
Organizational characteristics	• Organizational forms (what is the degree of economies of scale and scope and what are contractual relationships?) • Incentive regime (what is the degree of decision rights, market exposure, financial responsibility, accountability, and coverage of social functions?) • Linkages (what is the degree of horizontal and vertical integration or fragmentation?)
Institutional characteristics	• Stewardship (who controls strategic and operational decisions?) • Governance (what are the ownership arrangements?) • Insurance markets (what are the rules on revenue collection, pooling, and transfer of funds?) • Factor and product markets (from whom to buy, at what price, and how much?)

Source: Preker, Harding, and Travis (2000).

Figure 8A.1 Structure of Health Care Sources and Uses

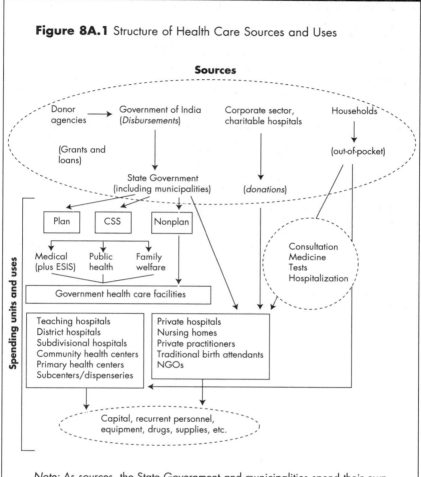

Note: As sources, the State Government and municipalities spend their own revenues on health as well as passing through disbursements from the central government. "Plan" refers to funds coming from Ninth Plan allocations for development purposes; CSS, centrally sponsored schemes; ESIS, Employees State Insurance Scheme; NGOs, nongovernmental organizations.
Source: Adapted from Sharma, McGreevey, and Hotchkiss (2000).

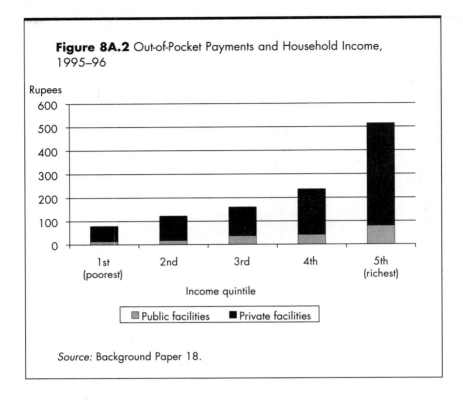

Figure 8A.2 Out-of-Pocket Payments and Household Income, 1995–96

Source: Background Paper 18.

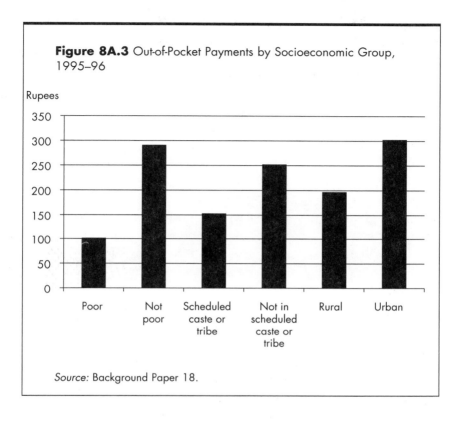

Figure 8A.3 Out-of-Pocket Payments by Socioeconomic Group, 1995–96

Source: Background Paper 18.

Notes

1. Data and analysis of resource allocation within the public sector and by households in the private sector are also presented in chapter 7.

2. The most recent source of detailed private spending on health is the 1995–96 National Sample Survey (National Sample Survey Organisation 1998) .

3. In keeping with standardized accounting methods for national health accounts, government expenditures on health-related areas of food distribution, water, and sanitation have been excluded from these estimates. Central and state government spending on health and family welfare is included.

4. Centrally financed services address different elements of the health sector (chapter 7).

5. Taxation in India is widely assumed to be progressive (Garg 2001), but detailed analytical work on the question is not available.

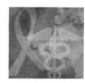 CHAPTER 9

Health System Outcomes

This chapter reviews the current state of health systems outcomes in India according to the health system objectives laid out in chapter 1:

- Improve the *health status* of the population by lowering mortality and morbidity rates

- Protect the population against the *financial risks* of health problems

- Respond to *citizens' demands and needs.*

Improving the health status of the population is often considered to be the most important objective of the health system, but the previously neglected areas of financial protection and health system responsiveness are also important; indeed they become critical for India as it moves into the health transition. Therefore, we analyze outcomes for all three objectives. We hope that in doing so we will stimulate a careful and transparent monitoring of the results of the health system, better planning for future interventions, and greater efficiency, equity, and public accountability in the health sector. See box 9.1 for a summary of the empirical findings and policy challenges discussed in the chapter.

Box 9.1 Empirical Findings and Policy Challenges

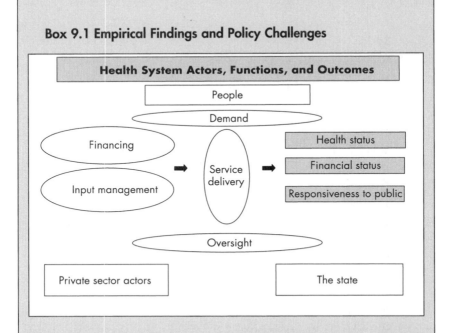

Health System Actors, Functions, and Outcomes

People

Demand

Financing

Input management

Service delivery

Health status

Financial status

Responsiveness to public

Oversight

Private sector actors

The state

Empirical Findings

Health Status
- Despite large gains in health status since independence, the poor continue to suffer widely from readily curable or preventable conditions—"the unfinished agenda" in world health. The poorest quintile of Indians have more than double the mortality rates, malnutrition, and fertility of the richest quintile.
- Disadvantaged groups in India—scheduled tribes and castes—have consistently worse health outcomes than other groups. Females also do worse in many health outcomes, as do people living in rural areas.
- Because the country bears a large share of the world's disease burden, progress toward global targets for diseases

of the unfinished agenda depends on increased action in India.

- With rising life expectancy, changing lifestyles, and progress in addressing the unfinished agenda, the epidemiological profile of India will shift increasingly toward diseases with higher costs per episode. The top causes of premature death and disability in India reflect this transition: (a) acute lower respiratory infections, (b) diarrheal diseases, (c) ischemic heart disease, (d) injuries from falls, and (e) major depression. Persistently high rates of maternal mortality and morbidity are linked to high fertility levels.
- There is no unique "Indian" health status but rather a diversity of state-level situations. Health conditions in Kerala are comparable to those in upper-middle-income countries such as Trinidad, Argentina, and Mauritius. Most Indian states, however, are comparable to lower-middle-income countries such as Brazil, Egypt, and Peru. Conditions in the poorest performing states are similar to those in low-income countries such as Sudan, Nigeria, and Tanzania.

Financial Protection

- The lack of prepayment systems for health care has put Indians at great financial risk in the event of hospitalization, and most of their total expenditures are in fact for hospitalization. About one-fourth of hospitalized Indians fall below the poverty line as a result of their hospital stays. The use of public hospitals reduces this risk only marginally.
- Financial risk from serious illness affects nearly all income groups in India, with more than 40 percent of hospitalized patients depending on loans and the sale of assets to pay for hospitalization.

Box 9.1 (continued)

- Cost remains a significant barrier to the use of health care, particularly for the poor, who cannot afford the level or quality of care they need. Cost is a greater barrier than physical access to health providers.

Responsiveness to the Public
- India has a comprehensive set of laws, but mechanisms for enforcement of those laws and for the redress of patients' complaints function poorly, whether at the facility level, in consumer forums, or in the civil and criminal courts. These mechanism are in any case largely inaccessible to the poor, who require intermediaries for protection and meaningful voice.
- Users of the public hospitals are less satisfied than those in the private sector. Women who use public health facilities express concerns about lack of privacy, lack of female doctors, lack of confidentiality, and long waiting times to see a doctor. In Andhra Pradesh and Uttar Pradesh, specific areas of dissatisfaction include the cost of services (particularly unofficial payments for nominally free services and drugs), lack of cleanliness of facilities, and behavior of health staff.

Policy Challenges
- How can the health system be made more pro-poor, gender-sensitive, and client-friendly to respond to the high burden of preventable disease borne by the poor, women, and scheduled tribes and castes?
- How can India strengthen financing systems to reduce the large financial risks faced by Indians, particularly the poor, when they become ill? As the burden of disease

shifts toward diseases with a high cost per episode, this challenge becomes more pressing.

- How can the experience of stronger states be replicated in weaker performing states to improve health status and reduce polarization?
- How can new and more responsive mechanisms be put in place to protect consumer interests and increase social accountability of the health system? In addition to better enforcement of existing laws, can other approaches be used, such as promoting consumer rights, increasing public awareness of health and consumer issues, and enhancing the voice of the poor?

Health Status

We begin the analysis of health status outcomes by comparing India's health burden with that of the world and then examine India's trends in mortality, fertility, malnutrition, and illness. We also focus on disparities in health status within India, looking at differences between states, sexes, the poor, and scheduled castes and tribes.

India's Share of the World's Health Problems

India carries a large burden of the world's disease, as one would expect given its large population and high levels of poverty (table 9.1 and appendix table 9A.1). India has a major portion of the world's child and maternal deaths as well as a disproportionate amount of the disease burden due to tuberculosis, leprosy, and immunizable diseases. Worldwide progress against these conditions will depend on India's achievements. Also, although India's burden of HIV infections is not disproportionate (14 percent of the world's cases), India will need to play a central role in preventing the further spread of the HIV/AIDS pandemic.

Table 9.1 India's Share of the World's Health Problems
(percent)

POPULATION	PEOPLE LIVING IN POVERTY (LESS THAN US$1/DAY)	TOTAL DEATHS	UNDER-FIVE MORTALITY (DEATHS PER 1,000 LIVE BIRTHS)	MATERNAL DEATHS
17	36	17	23	20

DALYS LOST	DEATHS PREVENTABLE WITH CHILDHOOD VACCINATIONS	HIV CASES	TUBERCULOSIS CASES	LEPROSY CASES
20	26	14	30	68

Note: DALYs, disability-adjusted life years.
Source: World Bank (2000d); WHO (2000c).

Although India's share of the world's deaths (appendix table 9A.2) is about equal to its share of the world's population (17 percent), the country's contribution to pre–health transition diseases affecting younger people is disproportionately high (table 9.2 and appendix table 9A.3). Compared with its share of the world's population, India has high levels of deaths due to traditional childhood infectious diseases such as acute lower respiratory infections (pneumonia), diarrhea, measles, and tetanus. These conditions, as well as tuberculosis—another disease with a high death rate in India—are common to low-income countries at the early stages of an epidemiological transition. However, India's top cause of death, ischemic heart disease (which results in heart attacks), is a condition of adulthood that becomes an increasing burden in countries already undergoing an epidemiological transition. Heart disease deaths are already relatively more common in India than in the rest of the world, despite the younger age structure of the country's population. Road traffic injury is the sixth most common cause of death in India and is also more frequent in India than in the rest of the world.

A fuller measure of the burden of disease counts not only deaths but also years of healthy life lost due to disability. A consolidated measure of losses from death and disability is disability-adjusted life

Table 9.2 Top 10 Specific Causes of Death in India, 1998

	INDIA		INDIA'S PERCENTAGE OF WORLDWIDE
CAUSE OF DEATH	NUMBER (THOUSANDS)	PERCENT	CASES
Ischemic heart disease	1,471	15.8	19.9
Acute lower respiratory infections	969	10.4	28.1
Diarrheal diseases	711	7.6	32.1
Cerebrovascular disease	557	6.0	10.9
Tuberculosis	421	4.5	28.1
Road traffic injury	217	2.3	18.5
Measles	190	2.0	21.4
HIV/AIDS	179	1.9	7.8
Tetanus	165	1.8	40.3
Chronic obstructive pulmonary disease	153	1.6	6.8
Total deaths	9,337	100.0	17.3
Total population	982,223	100.0	16.7

Source: WHO (1999).

years (DALYs) lost. India's share of the world's total burden of DALYs lost was 19.5 percent, moderately larger than its 16.7 percent share of the world's population (table 9.3). Except for depression, India's contributions to all leading causes of DALYs lost are greater than its proportion of the world's population. Diseases characteristic of the pre–health transition still figure prominently in India, particularly childhood infections (pneumonia, diarrhea, and measles), as well as tuberculosis and anemia. However, other conditions are also significant. Injuries from falls, road traffic accidents, and fires each account for relatively large portions of DALYs lost in India—and in comparison to the rest of the world. Ischemic heart disease and depression also make up a large burden of disease in India, ranking third and fifth respectively among specific causes of DALYs lost in India.

The World Health Organization (WHO 2000c) ranks India 134th of 191 countries in disability-adjusted life expectancy at birth. Although India's infant mortality and total fertility rates are near the average for low-income countries, it has relatively high levels of childhood malnutrition (appendix table 9A.3). Fortunately, India is not yet suffering from the low levels of disability-adjusted life

Table 9.3 Top 10 Specific Causes of DALYs Lost in India, 1998

CAUSE OF DALYS LOST	INDIA		
	NUMBER OF DALYs LOST	PERCENT	INDIA'S PERCENTAGE OF WORLD
Acute lower respiratory infections	24,806	9.2	30.1
Diarrheal diseases	22,005	8.2	30.1
Ischemic heart disease	11,697	4.3	22.5
Falls (injuries)	10,898	4.1	40.3
Unipolar major depression	9,679	3.6	16.6
Tuberculosis	7,577	2.8	26.9
Road traffic injuries	7,204	2.7	18.5
Measles	6,474	2.4	21.4
Anemia	6,302	2.3	25.5
Fire-related injuries	5,723	2.1	47.8
All causes	268,953	100.0	19.5
Population (thousands)	982,223	100.0	16.7

Note: DALYs, disability-adjusted life years.
Source: WHO (1999).

expectancy seen across Africa (including middle-income countries like South Africa), where the HIV epidemic is further advanced. Yet in a comparison of country performance of health outcomes between 1960 and 1990 (Wang and others 1999), India performed worse than predicted by its income and education levels in the areas of mortality of those under the age of five years, female adult mortality, and total fertility. India performed better than expected for male adult mortality.

National Health Status Trends

India's life expectancy has shown remarkable improvement, rising from 49 years in 1970 to 63 years in 1998. Similarly, infant mortality dropped from 146 deaths per 1,000 births in the 1950s to 70 in 1999, while the total fertility rate fell significantly, from 6.0 in the 1960s to 3.3 in 1999 (Registrar General 1999a, 2000). Little progress has been made since the mid-1990s, however, in the area of malnutrition. Although Indians no longer suffer from the waves of famine that marked earlier periods in the nation's history, recent surveys show that

47 percent of all children under three are underweight, down from 52 percent six years previously (IIPS 2000). In addition, nearly three-fourths of children under five are anemic, a condition that significantly harms cognitive development (IIPS 2000).

Despite the marked long-term reduction in infant mortality, the pace of India's infant mortality reduction, like its progress on malnutrition, has slowed during the 1990s (figure 9.1). Since the infant mortality rate is a sensitive indicator that responds to many underlying causes, including general socioeconomic conditions and the use of health services, the reasons for the slowdown are not obvious. One explanation lies in the coincident slowdown in poverty reduction over the same period (Kathuria and Hanson 2000). More immediate

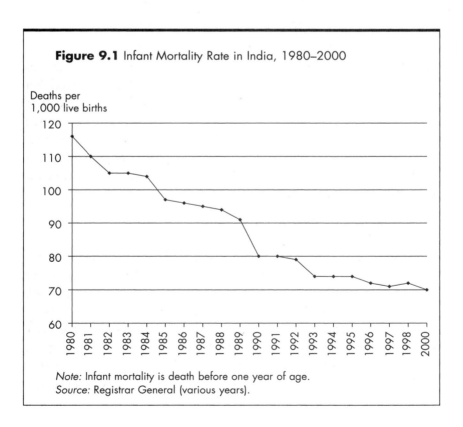

Figure 9.1 Infant Mortality Rate in India, 1980–2000

Deaths per
1,000 live births

Note: Infant mortality is death before one year of age.
Source: Registrar General (various years).

causes are related to the stubbornly high levels of malnutrition and disease; the latter is due in part to persistently high levels of exposure to disease combined with languishing rates of immunization coverage and low use of health services for safe motherhood and common diseases of infancy (Claeson, Bos, and Pathamanathan 1999).

The introduction of child survival initiatives in the 1980s—such as universal immunization and control of diarrheal disease and acute respiratory infections—may have made important contributions to the reduction of postneonatal mortality rates (from age one month to one year). Neonatal deaths now comprise the majority of infant deaths and may be attributed to poor maternity care, maternal malnutrition, and a high risk of neonatal infections (Ministry of Health and Family Welfare 2000b). National surveys show that about half of all women of reproductive age were anemic in 1998–99 and that only one-third of births were institutional deliveries (IIPS 2000). Each of these conditions contributes to high neonatal mortality.

Although the decline in adult mortality accelerated through the 1990s compared with previous decades, the rate of decline of child mortality was faster in the 1980s than it was in the 1970s or the 1990s. The annual rate of decline in mortality for children under five was 3.6 percent between 1981 and 1991, before dropping to 2.0 percent between 1991 and 1996. The same rate dropped by 2.1 percent per year between 1971 and 1981. Because India's population is young, reductions in overall death rates for India also slowed during the 1990s compared with the 1980s.

Overall death rates and DALYs lost appear to have dropped somewhat in the last decade (appendix table 9A.4), although part of the change may be due to differences in the measurement of mortality. Shifts in the composition of causes of death and disability appear to have accelerated over the 1990s. Chronic diseases of adulthood, notably heart disease and depression, as well as injuries, are playing an increasingly important role in India's burden of disease. HIV is also increasing at rapid rates. At the same time, India continues to have a high burden of readily preventable and treatable conditions due to childhood communicable diseases, tuberculosis, malnutrition, and maternal illness. These illnesses are concentrated in poorer states and among the poor.

Health Status Disparities

We have seen that the causes of death and disability are shifting rapidly in India while the overall levels of mortality and malnutrition are stabilizing at relatively high levels. In this section we will demonstrate how health outcomes are becoming increasingly polarized, first by providing some international comparisons of health outcomes and then by comparing health outcomes according to geographic region, gender, membership in scheduled castes and tribes, and poverty level.

International Comparisons

Both the average levels and inequality in health between the poor and better-off vary considerably from country to country (box 9.2). All countries show variations in health status—some people die in childhood while others survive to old age. Compared with many countries, however, India displays a high degree of variability in health status across its population. For example, India ranks 153rd of 191 countries in variability of child mortality (WHO 2000c). Estimates point to more variability in India than in China (ranked 101) and Bangladesh (ranked 125). India's variability of child mortality is similar to other low-income countries, like Ghana (ranked 149), Indonesia (ranked 156), and Nepal (ranked 161), but it is greater than that of Côte d'Ivoire (ranked 181), Pakistan (ranked 183), and Nigeria (ranked 188).

Health outcomes for women are generally worse than for men throughout the world; in India the disparity is more pronounced (World Bank 2000d). Although females are in the majority in most countries, only 48.4 percent of India's population is female, the eighth-lowest proportion in the world. Life expectancy at birth is usually considerably higher for females than males—4.1 years higher worldwide. However, the difference in India is only 1.5 years. Among 65 low- and middle-income countries for which data are available,

Box 9.2 "Achievement" Means Doing Well for *Everyone*—Not Just the Better-Off

Countries—and states within countries—typically vary both in average health and in the degree of inequality in health between the poor and better-off. For example, according to demographic and health surveys between 1990 and 1998, India had a lower under-five mortality rate than Bangladesh (119 compared with 128 per 1,000), but the inequality between the poor and the better-off was higher in India (Gwatkin and others 2000). A country's or state's "achievement" index captures both these considerations. Higher mortality rates among the poor push the achievement index (or, more correctly in this case, the *non*achievement index) above the sample mortality rate. The bigger the inequality by wealth, the greater the proportional "wedge" between achievement and the sample mean.

The simplest achievement index is the mean multiplied by the complement of the concentration index of inequality (Wagstaff 2002). The concentration index ranges from –1 (all mortality concentrated among the poorest), through 0 (all children have the same rate), to +1 (all mortality concentrated among the richest) (Kakwani and others 1997). To calculate the achievement index for under-five mortality, we take India's concentration index for under-five mortality, which is –0.17; find its complement, which means subtracting it from 1 (that is, 1 – (–0.17) = 1.17); and multiply the result by the under-five mortality rate (1.17 x 119 = 139). The final result is the achievement index for under-five mortality—139 per 1,000. By contrast, Bangladesh's concentration index is only –0.08, so its achievement index is 108 percent of 128, or 139 per 1,000—the same as India's, despite its higher average under-five mortality rate.

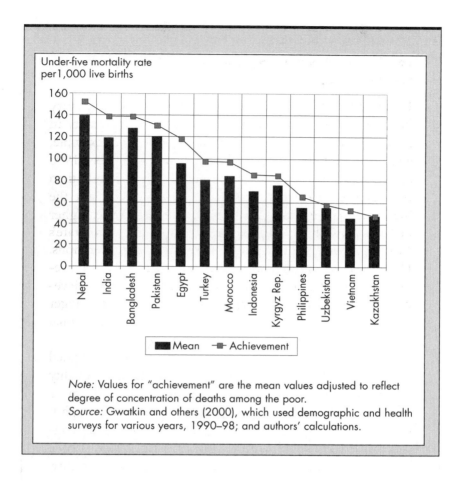

Under-five mortality rate
per 1,000 live births

■ Mean ──■── Achievement

Note: Values for "achievement" are the mean values adjusted to reflect degree of concentration of deaths among the poor.
Source: Gwatkin and others (2000), which used demographic and health surveys for various years, 1990–98; and authors' calculations.

India has the sixth-largest difference between female and male child mortality rates—13 deaths per 1,000 births.

Geographic Disparity

Disparities in India are also reflected in the large and growing inter-state differentials in infant mortality (appendix table 9A.5). In 1998, infant mortality rates were as high as 98 per 1,000 live births in Orissa and Madhya Pradesh, 85 in Uttar Pradesh, and 83 in Rajasthan (Registrar General 1999b). At the other end of the spectrum, Kerala had a remarkably low rate (16), followed by Maharashtra (49), Tamil Nadu (53), Punjab (54), and Karnataka (58). Within states, large differences appear between districts, with the worst-off districts found in states with the poorest overall mortality rates. Urban areas consistently have better health outcomes than rural areas, although these figures probably conceal the extent of poor health in urban and periurban slums, where many migrants live and where few organized primary health services are available.

Fertility rates also vary widely among the states (see appendix table 9A.5). These differences are significant not only because they prompt different strategies for fertility reduction in different states but also because population shifts have important implications for changes in the division of public resources and political representation. Only two of the fifteen major states have reached so-called replacement levels of fertility (where the total fertility rate is no greater than 2.1 births per woman aged 15 to 49). Another five major states have total fertility rates of between 2.1 and 3. However, in eight major states the rate is 3 or more; these states comprise about 44 percent of India's population and include the poorest states with the highest rates of infant mortality. The differences among states stem largely from poverty, illiteracy, and inadequate access to health and family welfare services (Ministry of Health and Family Welfare 2000b).

Interstate differences in malnutrition are also noteworthy (appendix table 9A.6). In a pattern consistent with the synergistic relationship between illness and malnutrition, the states known to have poor mortality outcomes also have higher levels of malnutrition. Even in the states with the lowest levels of malnutrition (Kerala and Punjab), more than one-fourth of children below three years of age are still malnourished. While the situation in Punjab and Haryana is no doubt improved by fertile and irrigated land, Assam has relatively low levels of malnutrition despite its relative lack of the endowments enjoyed by Punjab and Haryana.

To assess changes in state levels of malnutrition over time, we examined the results of two rounds of the National Family Health Survey (IIPS 2000). During the six years between the two rounds (1992–93

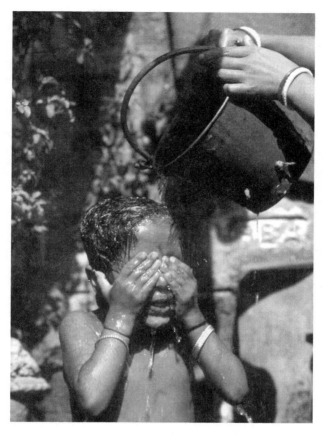

A refreshing shower (PHOTOGRAPH BY RAY WITLIN/THE WORLD BANK PHOTO LIBRARY)

and 1998–99), levels of severe and total malnutrition (6.4 percent) have declined only marginally among children under three in India (to 2.6 percent and 6.4 percent respectively), according to measures of weight for age (appendix table 9A.7). Malnutrition levels are estimated to have increased between the rounds in Rajasthan, Haryana, and Madhya Pradesh; all other states have shown varying amounts of improvement. The largest gains in child nutrition status were observed in the states of Punjab, Assam, Tamil Nadu, Andhra Pradesh, and Karnataka, all of which improved by more than 10 percentage points.

The high level of diversity in under-five mortality between and within states can make national measures highly misleading from a policy point of view. Some states compare well with middle-income countries, whereas others fare much worse (table 9.4). Kerala is a clear outlier—its under-five mortality rate is comparable to that of upper-middle-income countries such as Trinidad, Argentina, and Mauritius. The rate in most Indian states, by contrast, is comparable to that in lower-middle-income countries such as Brazil, Egypt, and Peru. The poorest-performing states compare with poor countries such as Sudan, Nigeria, and Tanzania. The Indian average rate

Table 9.4 Under-Five Mortality Rates in Indian States and in the World

UNDER-FIVE MORTALITY RATE BY COUNTRY INCOME GROUP (DEATHS PER 1,000 LIVE BIRTHS)	INDIAN STATE	INTERNATIONAL COMPARISON
Upper-middle-income countries		
Less than 20	Kerala	Trinidad, Uruguay, Argentina, Mauritius
Lower-middle-income countries		
40–50	Himachal Pradesh, Goa	Brazil, Tunisia, Peru, Dominican Republic
50–65	Mizoram, Delhi, Manipur, Maharashtra, Tamil Nadu, Nagaland	Guatemala, Egypt, Morocco
65–80	West Bengal, Karnataka, Sikkim, Punjab, Haryana	Papua New Guinea, Bolivia
Low-income countries		
80–100	Jammu and Kashmir, Gujarat, Andhra Pradesh, Assam, Arunachal Pradesh	Benin, Yemen
100–140	Orissa, Bihar, Rajasthan, Meghalaya, Uttar Pradesh, Madhya Pradesh	Sudan, Nigeria, Zimbabwe, Tanzania
Greater than 140	No Indian State	Angola, Cameroon, Ethiopia, Malawi, Mali, Uganda, Zambia

Note: Under-five mortality is measured from birth up to five years of age.
Source: Data for Indian states are from IIPS (2000). Data for countries are from World Bank (2000d).

for under-five mortality is now 94.9, a level considerably higher than the average of 79 for low- and middle-income countries.

Gender Disparity

As noted above, gender disparity in health outcomes is particularly prominent in India. India has approximately 933 females to every 1,000 males and has had that low ratio for more than 30 years.[1] The largest gender disparities in India are found in the northern states, notably Haryana and Punjab, despite their relative prosperity. Among Indian states, only Kerala had more women than men in 2001. The low ratio of women to men is usually attributed to a preference for sons, discrimination against girls (which results in lower female literacy, among other things), female feticide, and higher mortality levels among females (Ministry of Health and Family Welfare 2000b).

Girls start out having lower mortality rates than do boys during the first month of life (the neonatal period), which accounts for their lower rates of infant mortality (that is, death in the first year of life) (appendix table 9A.8). However, death rates in the postneonatal period (age one month to one year) and in the whole period up to age five (under-five mortality), are higher for girls (IIPS 2000). Girls have higher childhood mortality despite the fact that boys are reported to have a higher prevalence of acute respiratory infections and similar levels of diarrhea and anemia—major causes of childhood death. This paradox may be explained by the fact that boys are more likely to receive health care: 66.5 percent of boys with acute respiratory infections are taken to a health provider, compared with 60.8 percent of girls (IIPS 2000). Girls also have marginally higher rates of malnutrition, which places them at higher risk of severe illness and death.

In contrast to childhood illnesses, the prevalence of medically treated tuberculosis is significantly lower among females than males (appendix table 9A.8), which is also the case in most of the world. The possible reasons are that males are more likely to come into contact with tuberculosis or simply have a higher susceptibility, though it has also been suggested that their higher smoking rates may also contribute (IIPS 2000).

The relative neglect of women's health is also reflected in poor reproductive health indicators: maternal mortality is estimated at over 407 deaths per 100,000 live births in India (Registrar General 2000), compared with an average of 350 among low- and middle-income countries (World Bank 1997a). A major reason for the poor maternal health outcomes are the high levels of malnutrition among women. In 1998–99, 52 percent of all women of reproductive age were found to be anemic, and 36 percent were chronically malnourished (IIPS 2000). Low levels of access to, and utilization of, safe motherhood services could also contribute to higher maternal mortality.

Scheduled Castes and Tribes

Data on health outcomes among scheduled castes and tribes show consistently that these groups are at a disadvantage (table 9.5). Of all disadvantaged groups in India, scheduled tribes tend to have the highest rates of infant and child mortality, malnutrition, and morbidity, followed by scheduled castes and then by other disadvantaged (or "backward") classes. Total fertility rates are highest among scheduled castes.

Poverty Disparity

Large-scale studies that assess specific causes of illness and death by level of poverty are not available in India. Yet India continues to suffer disproportionately from communicable diseases, malnutrition, and maternal conditions, which constitute the "unfinished agenda" of the health transition (Murray and Lopez 1996; World Bank 1997b). These conditions are concentrated among the poor (Gwatkin and others 2000). Compared with the poor, the rich are sick less, become sick at an older age, and suffer more from non-communicable diseases than from communicable diseases.

Examination of health status outcomes for Indians grouped according to wealth shows that the poor have much higher levels of mortal-

Table 9.5 Health Outcomes among Scheduled Castes, Tribes, and Rest of Population in India, 1998–99

OUTCOME	SCHEDULED CASTES	SCHEDULED TRIBES	OTHER DISADVANTAGED CLASSES	REST OF POPULATION
Infant mortality (per 1,000 births)	83.0	84.2	76.0	61.8
Under-five mortality (per 1,000 births)	119.3	126.6	103.1	82.6
Total fertility rate	3.15	3.06	2.83	2.66
Children underweight (percent)	53.5	55.9	47.3	41.1
Children with anemia (percent)[a]	78.3	79.8	72.0	72.7
Children with acute respiratory infection, during two-week period (percent)[a]	19.6	22.4	19.1	18.7
Children with diarrhea, during two-week period (percent)[a]	19.8	21.1	18.3	19.1
Anemia among women (percent)	56.0	64.9	50.7	47.6

Note: Infant mortality is of those less than one year of age; under-five mortality is of those less than five years of age; total fertility rate is lifetime births per woman ages 15–49; underweight children are those under three years of age whose weight is low for their age (that is, statistically below normal by more than 2 standard deviations).
a. Children under age three.
Source: IIPS (2000).

ity, malnutrition, and fertility than do the rich (table 9.6). Compared with the richest quintile, the poorest quintile generally had double the risks of infant and child death, malnutrition, and high fertility.

Although data from the most recent round of the National Family Health Survey are not yet available for direct comparison of trends among poverty quintiles (as was done with the 1992–93 survey), some early results show similar trends. Indians classified as having a low living standard suffer worse health outcomes than do those

Table 9.6 Health Status Indicators—Comparison between the Poorest and Richest Quintiles of the Indian Population, 1992–93

INDICATOR	POOREST QUINTILE (1)	RICHEST QUINTILE (2)	RISK RATIO (1) / (2)
Infant mortality (per 1,000 births)	109	44	2.5
Under-five mortality (per 1,000 births)	155	54	2.8
Underweight children (percent)	60	34	1.7
Total fertility rate	4.1	2.1	2.0

Note: For definitions of indicators, see general note to table 9.5.
Source: Gwatkin and others (2000).

classified as having a medium or high living standard (table 9.7). In particular, those from the low-standard-of-living group had more than double the rates of infant and child mortality and childhood malnutrition than the high-standard-of-living group. They also had 60 percent higher fertility rates, 34 percent more childhood acute respiratory infections, and 24 percent more childhood diarrhea. The smallest difference was for children with anemia: all groups had high levels, ranging from 67 percent to 79 percent.

Many pretransition diseases are concentrated among poor states and among poorer districts within states. For example, the poorest states in India account for 70 percent of the leprosy cases but for only 46 percent of the total population.[2] Equity analysis in these states confirms that the most socially vulnerable groups (scheduled castes and women below the poverty line) shoulder the highest burden of the disease (World Bank 2001). In Bihar, for example, prevalence rates for leprosy were 50 percent higher than the state average for men and women below the poverty line. The prevalence rate for scheduled castes is even higher—twice the state average. In Uttar Pradesh and Orissa, prevalence rates for scheduled castes are 2 to 2.5 times that of the state average. In West Bengal, prevalence rates for women below the poverty line were 4 times the state average.

Malaria has also been shown to be more prevalent in rural districts that have higher levels of illiteracy and larger populations of scheduled tribes (World Bank 1997c). Tuberculosis rates are highest

Table 9.7 Health Outcomes by Standard of Living, 1998–99

OUTCOME	STANDARD OF LIVING			RATIO, LOW TO HIGH
	LOW	MEDIUM	HIGH	
Infant mortality (per 1,000 births)	88.8	70.3	42.7	2.08
Under-five mortality (per 1,000 births)	130.0	94.6	51.5	2.52
Total fertility rate	3.37	2.85	2.10	1.60
Children underweight (percent)	56.9	46.8	26.8	2.12
Children with anemia (percent)[a]	78.7	73.5	67.3	1.17
Children with acute respiratory infection, during two-week period (percent)[a]	21.0	19.4	15.7	1.34
Children with diarrhea, during two-week period (percent)[a]	19.9	19.7	16.1	1.24
Anemia among women (percent)	60.2	50.3	41.9	1.44

Note: For definitions of outcomes, see notes to table 9.5.
a. Children under age three.
Source: IIPS (2000).

in poorer households living in crowded conditions. Maternal deaths are also found more frequently in poorer states (Registrar General 2000). Yet to label some diseases as diseases of the poor and others as diseases of the rich would be simplistic. Although communicable diseases, malnutrition, and maternal conditions are concentrated among the poor, they are not the only diseases that beset the poor. Chapter 7 reports that poorer Indians already have higher rates of ischemic heart disease and hypertension than more affluent Indians, and have higher prevalence of alcohol and tobacco use, important risk factors for noncommunicable diseases. The poor at all ages have a higher risk of getting virtually all diseases and of having worse outcomes (Frank and Mustard 1994).

Financial Protection

Health care financing matters for two reasons. First, it influences how much and what type of health care people receive when they fall ill, which in turn influences their ability to maintain and improve their health. In other words, health financing affects access to and use of health services. Second, health care financing influences the ability of a household to maintain its living standards when one of its members needs health care. This is the issue of *financial protection.* Consultations with the poor in India (Narayan and others 2000) revealed that, after illiteracy and unemployment, spending on health care was the greatest precursor to poverty among poor households and the greatest impediment to continued household solvency.

This section examines how financial protection in health operates in India, focusing on differences among Indians at different income levels. More specific assessments of health financing functions and how they influence financial protection are examined in chapter 8 and in the discussion of policy options in chapter 3. In addition to examining the issue of financial protection, this section also examines the other side of the coin—the effect of health financing arrangements on access to and use of health services.

Financial Protection and Progressivity

On average, about 5.3 percent of annual household expenditure in India is spent on health care, or about 13.7 percent of nonfood expenditures. As a proportion of nonfood expenditure, richer Indians spend marginally more than poorer Indians on health care, so the distribution of out-of-pocket health expenditures may be considered progressive (figure 9.2).[3] One reason is the linking of fees to a patient's income. According to the 1995–96 NSSO survey, fees paid at government health facilities have been very progressive, with the richest quintile of Indians paying 73 percent of the fees and the poorest quintile only 1.4 percent (Background Paper 5). However, these fees do not represent a significant portion of the actual costs of care, and not all the direct costs of illness are captured at public facilities. Moreover, most out-of-pocket expenditures from a hospital-ization do not go to the public hospital; diagnostic tests, drugs, materials, and other items often have to be purchased separately. In the private sector, too, fees are often charged on a progressive slid-ing scale, with the poor paying less. In Andhra Pradesh and Uttar Pradesh, nearly all private providers offer some level of free or dis-counted care to the poor (chapter 6).

The other main source of health revenue is taxation, which is assumed to be highly progressive in India. Overall, then, payments for health care are progressive. Viewed in this way, the fairness of financing might not seem to be a major issue in India. However, we also need to examine the effect of health financing on poverty and access to services.

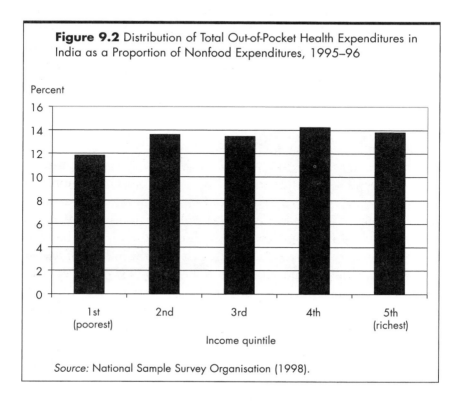

Figure 9.2 Distribution of Total Out-of-Pocket Health Expenditures in India as a Proportion of Nonfood Expenditures, 1995–96

Percent

Income quintile

Source: National Sample Survey Organisation (1998).

Financial Protection and Its Effect on Poverty

The fact that out-of-pocket payments are progressive simply means that they do not worsen the distribution of income. It says nothing about their effect on poverty. Spending even 4 percent of household income (or 12 percent of nonfood expenditures) on out-of-pocket payments represents a large drop in living standards for a low-income household and may make the difference between being just able to manage and falling into poverty.

The evidence suggests that the very large out-of-pocket payments in India do indeed leave people at great risk of financial catastrophe in the case of serious illness. Analysis of the NSSO data shows that the cost of a hospitalization for nearly all people is extremely high when compared with their total annual expenditures, averaging 58 percent. Although the richest 20 percent of Indians pay the highest proportion, they are not the most financially vulnerable. The rich have more resources to pay for their health care, whereas the poor lack savings, assets, income, and the ability to borrow at low interest to pay for health care, forcing them deeper into poverty when they get seriously ill.

An analysis of sources of financing for hospitalization shows that large proportions of all people borrow money or sell assets to pay for hospitalization (40 percent), but that doing so is more common among the bottom four income quintiles than among the richest, who are better able to use their current income and savings to finance hospitalization (figure 9.3). Further analysis shows that these trends hold for those hospitalized in both public and private hospitals, though the overall rate of borrowing and selling assets is about 5 percent lower in public hospitals.

The major states of India show large differences in the degree to which people below the poverty line finance hospitalization from borrowing or selling assets (figure 9.4). The data suggest high levels of borrowing for hospitalization in both the public and private sectors. Even though fees for public hospital admissions are minimal or nonexistent, hospitalization is still costly because patients often have to pay for diagnostic services or drugs, or because bribes are demanded. The data also indicate that the differences between states in the level of borrowing are larger than the differences between public and private sector hospitalizations within a state. That finding demonstrates that the failure to provide financial protection to the poor for the costs of hospitalization is significant across the country, even in the presence of public sector hospitals that provide nominally free care.

To learn how the costs of medical care might contribute to poverty levels in India, we used a conservative approach to calculate how many more people fell below the poverty line levels of consumption

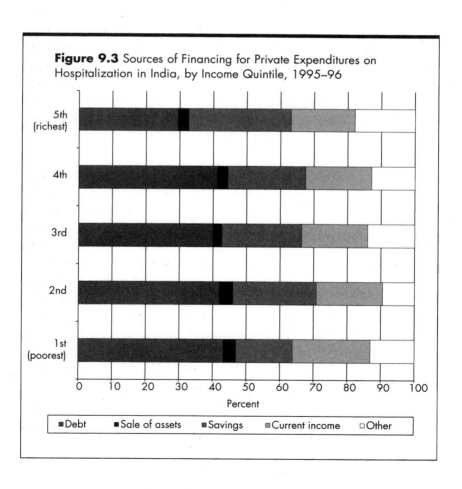

Figure 9.3 Sources of Financing for Private Expenditures on Hospitalization in India, by Income Quintile, 1995–96

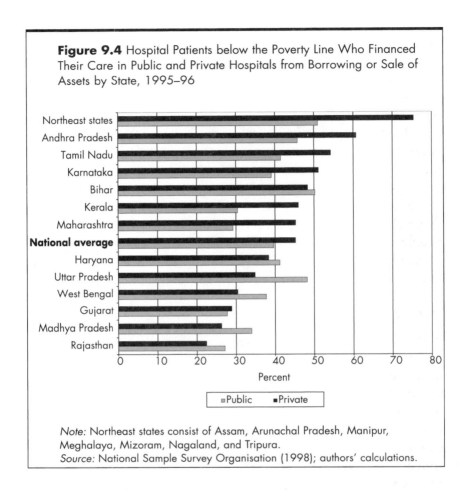

Figure 9.4 Hospital Patients below the Poverty Line Who Financed Their Care in Public and Private Hospitals from Borrowing or Sale of Assets by State, 1995–96

Percent

□ Public ■ Private

Note: Northeast states consist of Assam, Arunachal Pradesh, Manipur, Meghalaya, Mizoram, Nagaland, and Tripura.
Source: National Sample Survey Organisation (1998); authors' calculations.

after medical expenditures were eliminated from their consumption estimates. This analysis showed that direct out-of-pocket medical costs pushed 2.2 percent of Indians into poverty in one year.[4] Another way of looking at the same question is to determine the proportion of hospital patients who would fall below the poverty line after direct hospitalization costs were deducted. By this analysis, at least 24 percent of all people hospitalized in India in a single year fell below the poverty line because they were hospitalized. These estimates have limitations, as it is not clear how much people would consume if they did not have to pay for hospitalization. We nonetheless believe that the estimates may *underestimate* the effects of hospitalization on poverty because a large proportion of hospital spending was financed from borrowing, which is less likely to occur in the absence of serious illness.[5] Furthermore, the estimates include only the direct costs of medical care, which are less than the real costs of serious illness if lost earnings are also included.[6]

These quantitative estimates are reinforced by qualitative evidence (Narayan and others 2000). Households with sick and elderly people are reported to be invariably on the brink of ruin because of heavy expenditures for medical treatment. Lost wages and treatment expenses mean that poor groups are hit doubly hard by ill health.

Health Finance and Access to Health Services

The other side of the coin is the issue of whether the manner of health financing in India impedes access to and use of health services, and the evidence suggests that it does. The poor use health services less and do not have the same access to the facilities in the public or private sectors that are used by the better-off. (The question of who benefits from public and private health services is discussed in detail in chapter 7.) Furthermore, because the poor rely so widely on untrained health practitioners. the medical care they receive is of much lower *quality*.

The poor are less likely to seek care when ill (National Sample Survey Organisation 1998). On average, the poorest quintile of Indians is 2.6 times more likely than the richest to forgo medical treatment when ill. Aside from cases in which people believed that their illnesses were not serious (which comprised more than half of all cases), the main reason for not seeking care was cost, particularly for the poor (table 9.8).

By contrast, physical access to medical facilities was a much less common reason for not seeking care, although it too was strongly

Table 9.8 Indians Reporting an Illness within a 15-Day Period Who Did Not Seek Care, and Distribution of Reasons for Inaction, by Income Quintile, 1995–96

(percent)

BEHAVIOR AND REASONS	FIRST (POOREST)	SECOND	THIRD	FOURTH	FIFTH (RICHEST)	ALL	RATIO OF FIRST TO FIFTH QUINTILE
Did not seek care when ill	24.3	20.9	18.1	17.8	9.2	16.7	2.6
Distribution of reasons for not seeking care (percent of those not seeking care) Illness not considered serious	42.4	52.2	54.7	57.3	59.8	52.7	0.7
Cost	32.9	23.0	21.0	21.9	15.2	24.0	2.2
Medical facility not available in area	11.1	10.0	7.2	5.1	3.3	7.8	3.4
Other	13.6	14.4	16.6	15.2	21.7	15.6	0.6

Source: Background Paper 5; National Sample Survey Organisation (1998).

associated with poverty. The aggregate figures mask variations across and within states, as well as gender differences, but the overall relative importance of financial barriers to health care is similar across India.

Conclusions on Financing, Protection, and Access

The information on financial protection in India suggests that whereas overall financial contributions to health appear to be progressive, financial risk from serious illness affects nearly all income groups in India, with people from the four poorest quintiles depending on loans and sale of assets to pay for hospitalization. The lack of prepayment systems for health care has put Indians at great financial risk in the event of hospitalization, and most of their total expenditures are in fact spent on hospitalization. The use of public hospitals reduces this risk only marginally. Cost remains a significant barrier to the use of health care, particularly for the poor. Cost is a greater barrier than physical access to health providers.

Responsiveness to the Public

The final health system objective for which outcomes are examined in this chapter is that of responsiveness to the public, that is, how well the health system meets the expectations of the public (WHO 2000c).[7] Those expectations may include protection from fraud and abuse, respect, and satisfaction with service. Responsiveness is becoming increasingly important to politicians and public officials as the public comes increasingly to hold them accountable for public services. In the private sector, success depends in part on responsiveness to customers. For our analysis, we assessed responsiveness by looking at how consumers' interests are protected and how satisfied consumers are with the health services they receive.

Protecting Consumer Interests

The Indian Law Institute compiled rulings by courts and consumer forums on health issues to examine how well the law protected the health of citizens. It concluded that India has a comprehensive set of legal instruments. The courts have held that health is a fundamental right, as described in the Indian Constitution,[8] and have been active in defining the boundaries of medical negligence. The law is much stronger on paper than in practice, however, because of weak enforcement and long delays in judicial proceedings.

In part to respond to those problems, "consumer forums" were established under the Consumer Protection Act of 1986 to provide a quicker and less formal method to resolve public complaints. A study of the forums highlighted many inadequacies (Background Paper 10). The forums were rarely approached in medical negligence cases (except by well-educated men from forward castes) and were technically ill-prepared to deal with such cases. Ninety percent of cases required more than a year to reach a judgment, despite the legal requirement to pass judgment within 90 days.

The present study examined mechanisms of consumer redress at health facilities and found them to be poorly developed in both the public and private sectors (table 9.9).[9] Although most facilities claimed to have mechanisms such as complaint boxes, these often were absent or hard to find. Large public sector institutions tended to have formal mechanisms, whereas the private sector tended to do things more informally. Among the facilities that had systems for consumer complaints, the types of complaints most commonly received had to do with hospital amenities or billing issues rather than quality of clinical care, suggesting that consumers have little knowledge about medical services and low expectations of the care they receive.[10]

Table 9.9 Presence of Mechanisms of Consumer Redress at Public Health Facilities and Private Hospitals

(percent)

MECHANISM	PRIVATE FACILITIES		PUBLIC FACILITIES	
	30 OR MORE BEDS	FEWER THAN 30 BEDS	HOSPITALS	PRIMARY HEALTH CENTERS
Procedures or guidelines for receiving and processing complaints	25	10	20	0
Unit or individual responsible for settling disputes	79	43	67	67
Complaint box or book claimed	71	33	58	40
Complaint box or book observed	33	10	4	0

Source: Background Paper 10.

Client Satisfaction

Studies of client satisfaction with health services have only recently been introduced in India. One of the rare sources of national-level data on patient satisfaction comes from the NSSO 52nd round (NSSO 1998). The data suggest that the private health sector responds better to patient interests than does the public sector, a difference that may explain why the private sector is used more frequently than the public sector for most curative services and why it is growing. Across India, 44 percent of people using the private sector for outpatient care chose it because private doctors were more accessible than government doctors. Another 36 percent stated that they were less satisfied with treatment in the public sector, and 7 percent noted that medicines were not available in the public sector. As shown in figure 9.5, these opinions did not vary strongly when disaggregated by income.

Studies that directly measure patient satisfaction with health care are becoming an increasingly important tool for learning how health services might better respond to people's needs. Under the state health systems development projects, more such surveys are being used to monitor performance. To date they have been used for the most part to identify poorly performing hospitals and problem areas within hospitals.

Before a state health systems project was launched in Uttar Pradesh, a random-sample interview of more than 8,300 patients using public health services there showed fairly uniform levels of satisfaction (STEM 2000).[11] The item getting the lowest marks was the financial burden of health care, followed by the cleanliness of the facility. Access to the facility was quite satisfactory (96 percent satisfied), but satisfaction with availability of staff, perceived technical quality of care, and behavior of doctors and nurses was considerably lower. Interestingly, no major differences in opinions emerged between women and men or among castes. The widest differences in satisfaction were between the wealthiest and poorest quintiles regarding financial burden (19 percent-

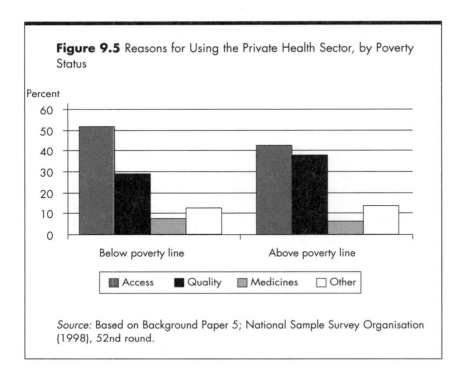

Figure 9.5 Reasons for Using the Private Health Sector, by Poverty Status

Source: Based on Background Paper 5; National Sample Survey Organisation (1998), 52nd round.

age point difference), availability of staff (12 percentage points), and behavior of nurses (9 percentage points). This disparity suggests not only that the poor in Uttar Pradesh are more bothered about the financial burden of health care in public facilities, but also that those with higher incomes are likely to be more satisfied with the staff and services, possibly because they are able to pay for better service.

Studies of satisfaction with private sector services explored differences in patient satisfaction between parts of the private and public sectors. In Andhra Pradesh, users of private facilities were consistently more satisfied with them than were users of public sector facilities, with the exception of nursing services used by the

Table 9.10 Patients Satisfied or Very Satisfied with Health Services in Public and Private Facilities in Andhra Pradesh, by Sex and Income Level (percent)

PATIENT/FACILITY	DIMENSION OF SATISFACTION						
	WAITING TIME	DOCTOR'S MANNER	DOCTOR'S SKILLS	NURSE'S MANNER	NURSE'S SKILLS	EXPLANATION OF CARE	OVERALL VISIT
Male							
Public	8.4	25.0	24.6	14.4	13.9	12.2	14.9
Private	12.7	42.6	41.2	16.3	15.3	16.7	28.1
Female							
Public	7.3	27.6	26.8	12.0	11.2	10.0	13.2
Private	16.6	46.3	43.7	14.0	13.1	16.0	25.1
Poorest quintile							
Public	10.0	23.8	24.4	21.2	21.6	14.6	20.4
Private	11.7	43.0	45.4	16.2	16.2	13.0	23.5
Richest quintile							
Public	5.5	30.3	24.8	9.3	8.4	17.4	8.4
Private	19.9	45.7	47.0	15.8	16.7	19.7	32.6
Total							
Public	7.8	26.4	25.8	13.2	12.5	11.0	14.0
Private	14.9	44.7	42.6	14.9	14.0	16.3	26.0

Source: Background Paper 20; authors' calculations.

poor (table 9.10).[12] Among users of private sector services, the richest quintile of Indians were more satisfied overall and more satisfied with waiting times than were the poorest quintile. Among users of public sector services, the rich tended to be more dissatisfied than the poor. Ratings by males and females were broadly similar.

Similar issues have emerged from a national survey of about 37,000 women asked about the quality of care on their most recent visit to a health facility (table 9.11). Public sector facilities were consistently rated lower than private facilities; the greatest amount of dissatisfaction involved the indicators for cleanliness, politeness, and privacy in the public sector facilities.

Table 9.11 Quality of Care Reported by Women after Their Most Recent Visit to a Health Facility, Public or Private, 1998–99
(percent)

INDICATOR OF CARE	PUBLIC SECTOR FACILITY	PRIVATE SECTOR FACILITY
Staff spent enough time	90.3	97.5
Staff talked nicely to them	62.7	78.4
Privacy was respected	68.2	83.9
Facility was very clean	52.1	75.3

Source: IIPS (2000).

Concluding Remarks

India bears a disproportionate amount of the world's disease burden. Moreover, India's disease profile is changing. High levels of pre-transition diseases persist as reductions in infant mortality and malnutrition slow their pace; at the same time, noncommunicable diseases and injuries are playing a growing role in the death and disability of Indians.

Our analysis of disparities in health outcomes showed a large polarization of conditions within India. Interstate differences appear to be widening, with wealthier states and states in the south improving at more rapid rates than poor and northern states. Individuals in scheduled tribes and castes are worse off, and women have worse outcomes than men in some respects. Finally, we showed that poverty is associated with many different types of poor health across India.

Our investigation of the responsiveness of the Indian health system to public concerns showed significant gaps in consumer protection and satisfaction. The poor appear to be at a disadvantage in both respects. The public and private sectors respond to consumers differentially, a subject examined in detail in chapter 6. Many improvements in responsiveness would not necessarily cost much money, but management attention and a public spotlight would be required to bring them about. Such improvements would likely contribute to more sustainable health services and improved utilization.

The general lack of some social means of insuring against the costs of health care in India needs to be corrected. The lack of insurance exacerbates inequities in health services and leaves the seriously ill financially vulnerable, even if they use the public health system. Addressing financial protection will require structural changes in the way health services are financed (chapter 8). However, such changes must also lead to improvements in quality and equity, which will contribute in turn to better health.

Appendix

Table 9A.1 Distribution of DALYs Lost in World, India, and Countries Grouped by Income, by Condition, 1998

CONDITION	WORLD NUMBER (THOUSANDS)	PERCENT	HIGH-INCOME COUNTRIES NUMBER (THOUSANDS)	PERCENT	LOW- AND MIDDLE-INCOME COUNTRIES NUMBER (THOUSANDS)	PERCENT	INDIA TOTAL NUMBER (THOUSANDS)	PERCENT	PERCENTAGE OF WORLD	PERCENTAGE LOW- AND MIDDLE-INCOME COUNTRIES
Memo: Distribution of population	5,884,576	100	907,828	15.4	4,976,748	84.6	982,223	100	16.7	19.7
All conditions	1,382,564	100	108,305	100	1,274,259	100	268,953	100	19.5	21.1
I. Communicable diseases, maternal and perinatal conditions, and nutritional deficiencies	565,528	40.9	7,834	7.2	557,694	43.8	135,263	50.3	23.9	24.3
A. Infectious and parasitic diseases	323,993	23.4	2,994	2.8	321,000	25.2	67,619	25.1	20.9	21.1
1. Tuberculosis	28,189	2.0	142	0.1	28,047	2.2	7,577	2.8	26.9	27.0
2. STDs excluding HIV	17,082	1.2	416	0.4	16,666	1.3	4,909	1.8	28.7	29.5
a. Syphilis	4,967	0.4	10	0.0	4,957	0.4	1,449	0.5	29.2	29.2
b. Chlamydia	7,150	0.5	354	0.3	6,796	0.5	1,982	0.7	27.7	29.2
c. Gonorrhea	4,955	0.4	46	0.0	4,909	0.4	1,479	0.5	29.8	30.1
d. Other STDs	10	0.0	5	0.0	5	0.0	0	0.0	0.0	0.0
3. HIV/AIDS	70,930	5.1	1,022	0.9	69,907	5.5	5,611	2.1	7.9	8.0
4. Diarrheal diseases	73,100	5.3	359	0.3	72,742	5.7	22,005	8.2	30.1	30.3
5. Childhood diseases	56,855	4.1	396	0.4	56,459	4.4	14,463	5.4	25.4	25.6

a. Pertussis	13,226	1.0	179	0.2	13,047	1.0	2,692	1.0	20.4	20.6
b. Poliomyelitis	213	0.0	0	0.0	213	0.0	63	0.0	29.4	29.4
c. Diphtheria	181	0.0	0	0.0	181	0.0	75	0.0	41.1	41.1
d. Measles	30,255	2.2	188	0.2	30,067	2.4	6,474	2.4	21.4	21.5
e. Tetanus	12,979	0.9	29	0.0	12,950	1.0	5,160	1.9	39.8	39.8
6. Meningitis	4,725	0.3	154	0.1	4,571	0.4	1,191	0.4	25.2	26.1
7. Hepatitis	1,700	0.1	55	0.1	1,645	0.1	300	0.1	17.7	18.3
8. Malaria	39,267	2.8	0	0.0	39,267	3.1	577	0.2	1.5	1.5
9. Tropical diseases	10,984	0.8	6	0.0	10,977	0.9	3,204	1.2	29.2	29.2
a. Trypanosomiasis	1,219	0.1	0	0.0	1,219	0.1	0	0.0	0.0	0.0
b. Chagas disease	589	0.0	0	0.0	588	0.0	0	0.0	0.0	0.0
c. Schistosomiasis	1,699	0.1	3	0.0	1,696	0.1	0	0.0	0.0	0.0
d. Leishmaniasis	1,710	0.1	3	0.0	1,707	0.1	1,141	0.4	66.8	66.9
e. lymphatic filariasis	4,698	0.3	0	0.0	4,698	0.4	2,063	0.8	43.9	43.9
f. Onchocerciasis	1,069	0.1	0	0.0	1,069	0.1	0	0.0	0.0	0.0
10. Leprosy	395	0.0	1	0.0	393	0.0	208	0.1	52.6	52.8
11. Dengue	558	0.0	0	0.0	558	0.0	353	0.1	63.2	63.2
12. Japanese encephalitis	503	0.0	0	0.0	502	0.0	66	0.0	13.1	13.1
13. Trachoma	1,263	0.1	8	0.0	1,255	0.1	32	0.0	2.5	2.6
14. Intestinal nematode infections	4,279	0.3	4	0.0	4,275	0.3	797	0.3	18.6	18.6
a. Ascariasis	1,292	0.1	1	0.0	1,290	0.1	163	0.1	12.6	12.6
b. Trichuriasis	1,287	0.1	0	0.0	1,287	0.1	102	0.0	7.9	7.9
c. Hookworm disease	1,698	0.1	2	0.0	1,695	0.1	532	0.2	31.3	31.4
d. Other intestinal infections	2	0.0	0	0.0	2	0.0	0	0.0	0.0	0.0

(Table continues on the following page.)

Table 9A.1 (continued)

CONDITION	WORLD		HIGH-INCOME COUNTRIES		LOW- AND MIDDLE-INCOME COUNTRIES		INDIA			
	NUMBER (THOUSANDS)	PERCENT	NUMBER (THOUSANDS)	PERCENT	NUMBER (THOUSANDS)	PERCENT	TOTAL NUMBER (THOUSANDS)	PERCENT	PERCENTAGE OF WORLD	PERCENTAGE LOW- AND MIDDLE-INCOME COUNTRIES
15. Other infectious diseases	14,163	1.0	430	0.4	13,734	1.1	6,325	2.4	44.7	46.1
B. Respiratory infections	85,085	6.2	1 488	1.4	83,597	6.6	25,556	9.5	30.0	30.6
1. Acute lower respiratory infections	82,344	6.0	1 355	1.3	80,990	6.4	24,806	9.2	30.1	30.6
2. Acute upper respiratory infections	975	0.1	50	0.0	924	0.1	274	0.1	28.2	29.7
3. Otitis media	1,766	0.1	84	0.1	1,683	0.1	475	0.2	26.9	28.2
C. Maternal conditions	32,250	2.3	398	0.4	31,852	2.5	7,891	2.9	24.5	24.8
1. Hemorrhage	3,833	0.3	25	0.0	3,807	0.3	902	0.3	23.5	23.7
2. Sepsis	5,965	0.4	49	0.0	5,916	0.5	1,338	0.5	22.4	22.6
3. Hypertensive disorders of pregnancy	1,882	0.1	18	0.0	1,865	0.1	441	0.2	23.4	23.6
4. Obstructed labor	7,040	0.5	250	0.2	6,790	0.5	1,601	0.6	22.7	23.6
5. Abortion	5,498	0.4	18	0.0	5,479	0.4	1,704	0.6	31.0	31.1
6. Other maternal conditions	8,032	0.6	37	0.0	7,995	0.6	1,905	0.7	23.7	23.8
D. Perinatal conditions	80,564	5.8	2,020	1.9	78,544	6.2	23,316	8.7	28.9	29.7
E. Nutritional deficiencies	43,636	3.2	935	0.9	42,701	3.4	10,881	4.0	24.9	25.5

1. Protein-energy malnutrition	14,931	1.1	122	0.1	14,810	1.2	3,734	1.4	25.0	25.2
2. Iodine deficiency	1,078	0.1	23	0.0	1,055	0.1	280	0.1	26.0	26.6
3. Vitamin A deficiency	2,801	0.2	8	0.0	2,793	0.2	565	0.2	20.2	20.2
4. Anemias	24,746	1.8	773	0.7	23,973	1.9	6,302	2.3	25.5	26.3
5. Other nutritional disorders	80	0.0	9	0.0	71	0.0	0	0.0	0.0	0.0
II. Noncommunicable conditions	595,363	43.1	87,732	81.0	507,631	39.8	88,657	33.0	14.9	17.5
A. Malignant neoplasms	80,837	5.8	16,257	15.0	64,580	5.1	8,754	3.3	10.8	13.6
1. Mouth and oropharynx	4,473	0.3	446	0.4	4,027	0.3	1,313	0.5	29.4	32.6
2. Esophagus	4,180	0.3	398	0.4	3,782	0.3	681	0.3	16.3	18.0
3. Stomach	8,156	0.6	1,049	1.0	7,107	0.6	615	0.2	7.5	8.6
4. Colon/rectum	5,191	0.4	1,818	1.7	3,373	0.3	307	0.1	5.9	9.1
5. Liver	7,878	0.6	391	0.4	7,486	0.6	176	0.1	2.2	2.4
6. Pancreas	1,761	0.1	669	0.6	1,092	0.1	102	0.0	5.8	9.4
7. Trachea/bronchus/lung	11,176	0.8	3,122	2.9	8,054	0.6	921	0.3	8.2	11.4
8. Melanoma and other skin cancers	611	0.0	264	0.2	347	0.0	18	0.0	3.0	5.3
9. Breast	5,202	0.4	1,643	1.5	3,560	0.3	711	0.3	13.7	20.0
10. Cervix	3,183	0.2	199	0.2	2,985	0.2	836	0.3	26.2	28.0
11. Corpus uteri	705	0.1	199	0.2	506	0.0	42	0.0	6.0	8.3
12. Ovary	1,545	0.1	403	0.4	1,142	0.1	206	0.1	13.3	18.0
13. Prostate	1,551	0.1	673	0.6	878	0.1	87	0.0	5.6	9.9
14. Bladder	1,392	0.1	429	0.4	963	0.1	77	0.0	5.6	8.0

(Table continues on the following page.)

Table 9A.1 (continued)

CONDITION	WORLD		HIGH-INCOME COUNTRIES		LOW- AND MIDDLE-INCOME COUNTRIES		INDIA TOTAL		PERCENTAGE OF WORLD	PERCENTAGE LOW- AND MIDDLE-INCOME COUNTRIES
	NUMBER (THOUSANDS)	PERCENT	NUMBER (THOUSANDS)	PERCENT	NUMBER (THOUSANDS)	PERCENT	NUMBER (THOUSANDS)	PERCENT		
15. Lymphoma	3,419	0.2	759	0.7	2,659	0.2	360	0.1	10.5	13.5
16. Leukaemia	4,828	0.3	630	0.6	4,198	0.3	429	0.2	8.9	10.2
17. Other cancers	15,586	1.1	3,164	2.9	12,421	1.0	1,874	0.7	12.0	15.1
B. Other neoplasms	4,032	0.3	880	0.8	3,152	0.2	238	0.1	5.9	7.6
C. Diabetes mellitus	11,668	0.8	3,131	2.9	8,537	0.7	1,981	0.7	17.0	23.2
D. Nutritional/endocrine disorders	5,804	0.4	1,217	1.1	4,588	0.4	96	0.0	1.7	2.1
E. Neuropsychiatric disorders	159,462	11.5	25,414	23.5	134,048	10.5	22,944	8.5	14.4	17.1
1. Unipolar major depression	58,246	4.2	7,029	6.5	51,217	4.0	9,679	3.6	16.6	18.9
2. Bipolar affective disorder	16,189	1.2	1,768	1.6	14,421	1.1	2,746	1.0	17.0	19.0
3. Psychoses	14,265	1.0	2,280	2.1	11,984	0.9	1,964	0.7	13.8	16.4
4. Epilepsy	5,147	0.4	488	0.5	4,659	0.4	936	0.3	18.2	20.1
5. Alcohol dependence	18,292	1.3	4,739	4.4	13,553	1.1	1,074	0.4	5.9	7.9
6. Alzheimer and other dementias	8,510	0.6	2,983	2.8	5,527	0.4	922	0.3	10.8	16.7
7. Parkinson's disease	1,109	0.1	489	0.5	621	0.0	138	0.1	12.4	22.2
8. Multiple sclerosis	1,530	0.1	221	0.2	1,308	0.1	234	0.1	15.3	17.8
9. Drug dependence	6,326	0.5	1,544	1.4	4,782	0.4	89	0.0	1.4	1.9
10. Post traumatic stress disorder	2,174	0.2	278	0.3	1,896	0.1	369	0.1	17.0	19.4

11. Obsessive-com- pulsive disorders	11,566	0.8	1,504	1.4	10,062	0.8	1,947	0.7	16.8	19.4
12. Panic disorders	5,429	0.4	719	0.7	4,710	0.4	882	0.3	16.2	18.7
13. Other neuro- psychiatric disorders	10,678	0.8	1,370	1.3	9,308	0.7	1,964	0.7	18.4	21.1
F. Sense organ disorders	12,542	0.9	158	0.1	12,385	1.0	3,701	1.4	29.5	29.9
1. Glaucoma	3,070	0.2	85	0.1	2,985	0.2	698	0.3	22.8	23.4
2. Cataracts	9,182	0.7	68	0.1	9,114	0.7	3,001	1.1	32.7	32.9
3. Other sense organ disorders	290	0.0	5	0.0	286	0.0	2	0.0	0.7	0.7
G. Cardiovascular diseases	143,015	10.3	19,518	18.0	123,497	9.7	26,932	10.0	18.8	21.8
1. Rheumatic heart disease	6,576	0.5	180	0.2	6,396	0.5	1,793	0.7	27.3	28.0
2. Ischemic heart disease	51,948	3.8	9,501	8.8	42,447	3.3	11,697	4.3	22.5	27.6
3. Cerebrovascular disease	41,626	3.0	5,219	4.8	36,407	2.9	4,814	1.8	11.6	13.2
4. Inflammatory cardiac disease	10,509	0.8	722	0.7	9,787	0.8	2,071	0.8	19.7	21.2
5. Other cardiac diseases	32,356	2.3	3,896	3.6	28,460	2.2	6,556	2.4	20.3	23.0
H. Respiratory diseases	61,603	4.5	8,050	7.4	53,553	4.2	5,833	2.2	9.5	10.9
1. Chronic obstruc- tive pulmonary disease	28,654	2.1	2,449	2.3	26,205	2.1	2,536	0.9	8.9	9.7
2. Asthma	10,968	0.8	1,208	1.1	9,760	0.8	1,525	0.6	13.9	15.6

(Table continues on the following page.)

Table 9A.1 (continued)

CONDITION	WORLD		HIGH-INCOME COUNTRIES		LOW- AND MIDDLE-INCOME COUNTRIES		INDIA			
							TOTAL			
	NUMBER (THOUSANDS)	PERCENT	NUMBER (THOUSANDS)	PERCENT	NUMBER (THOUSANDS)	PERCENT	NUMBER (THOUSANDS)	PERCENT	PERCENTAGE OF WORLD	PERCENTAGE LOW- AND MIDDLE- INCOME COUNTRIES
3. Other respiratory diseases	18,392	1.3	1,303	1.2	17,089	1.3	3,352	1.2	18.2	19.6
I. Digestive diseases	41,111	3.0	4,365	4.0	36,746	2.9	5,618	2.1	13.7	15.3
1. Peptic ulcer disease	2,637	0.2	241	0.2	2,395	0.2	853	0.3	32.4	35.6
2. Cirrhosis of the liver	12,813	0.9	1,638	1.5	11,175	0.9	2,628	1.0	20.5	23.5
3. Appendicitis	1,446	0.1	35	0.0	1,411	0.1	313	0.1	21.7	22.2
4. Other digestive diseases	24,216	1.8	2,451	2.3	21,765	1.7	1,823	0.7	7.5	8.4
J. Diseases of the genito-urinary system	15,576	1.1	1,220	1.1	14,356	1.1	2,036	0.8	13.1	14.2
1. Nephritis/ nephrosis	8,429	0.6	470	0.4	7,959	0.6	1,578	0.6	18.7	19.8
2. Benign prostatic hypertrophy	2,150	0.2	239	0.2	1,911	0.1	366	0.1	17.0	19.2
3. Other genito-urinary system diseases	4,997	0.4	511	0.5	4,486	0.4	92	0.0	1.8	2.0
K. Skin diseases	1,619	0.1	136	0.1	1,482	0.1	114	0.0	7.0	7.7
L. Musculoskeletal diseases	21,464	1.6	4,512	4.2	16,952	1.3	1,710	0.6	8.0	10.1
1. Rheumatoid arthritis	3,682	0.3	991	0.9	2 692	0.2	197	0.1	5.4	7.3

2. Osteoarthritis	15,513	1.1	3,046	2.8	12,468	1.0	1,482	0.6	9.6	11.9
3. Other musculo-skeletal diseases	2,269	0.2	476	0.4	1,793	0.1	31	0.0	1.4	1.7
M. Congenital abnormalities	28,147	2.0	1,915	1.8	26,232	2.1	7,454	2.8	26.5	28.4
N. Oral diseases	8,483	0.6	959	0.9	7,524	0.6	1,247	0.5	14.7	16.6
1. Dental caries	4,720	0.3	432	0.4	4,288	0.3	783	0.3	16.6	18.2
2. Periodontal disease	295	0.0	36	0.0	258	0.0	86	0.0	29.2	33.3
3. Edentulism	3,351	0.2	485	0.4	2,866	0.2	356	0.1	10.6	12.4
4. Other oral diseases	118	0.0	7	0.0	111	0.0	22	0.0	18.8	19.9
III. Injuries	221,673	16.0	12,739	11.8	208,934	16.4	45,032	16.7	20.3	21.6
A. Unintentional	156,184	11.3	8,972	8.3	147,213	11.6	39,716	14.8	25.4	27.0
1. Road traffic accidents	38,849	2.8	4,556	4.2	34,293	2.7	7,204	2.7	18.5	21.0
2. Poisoning	6,364	0.5	280	0.3	6,085	0.5	988	0.4	15.5	16.2
3. Falls	27,021	2.0	1,397	1.3	25,624	2.0	10,898	4.1	40.3	42.5
4. Fires	11,967	0.9	261	0.2	11,706	0.9	5,723	2.1	47.8	48.9
5. Drowning	14,896	1.1	280	0.3	14,616	1.1	2,703	1.0	18.1	18.5
6. Other unintentional injuries	57,088	4.1	2,198	2.0	54,890	4.3	12,201	4.5	21.4	22.2
B. Intentional	65,489	4.7	3,768	3.5	61,721	4.8	5,316	2.0	8.1	8.6
1. Self-inflicted	21,511	1.6	2,416	2.2	19,095	1.5	3,337	1.2	15.5	17.5
2. Homicide and violence	21,573	1.6	1,210	1.1	20,363	1.6	1,847	0.7	8.6	9.1
3. War	22,405	1.6	142	0.1	22,264	1.7	132	0.0	0.6	0.6

Note: STD, sexually transmitted disease.
Source: WHO (1999).

307

Table 9A.2 Distribution of Deaths in World, India, and Countries Grouped by Income, by Cause, 1998

CAUSE	WORLD NUMBER (THOUSANDS)	PERCENT	HIGH-INCOME COUNTRIES NUMBER (THOUSANDS)	PERCENT	LOW- AND MIDDLE-INCOME COUNTRIES NUMBER (THOUSANDS)	PERCENT	INDIA TOTAL NUMBER (THOUSANDS)	PERCENT	PERCENTAGE OF WORLD	PERCENTAGE LOW- AND MIDDLE-INCOME COUNTRIES
Memo: Distribution of population	5,884,576	100	907,828	15.4	4,976,748	84.6	982,223	100	16.7	19.7
Total Deaths	53,929	100	8,033	100	45,897	100	9,337	100	17.3	20.3
I. Communicable diseases, maternal and perinatal conditions, and nutritional deficiencies	16,447	30.5	510	6.3	15,937	34.7	3,944	42.2	24.0	24.7
A. Infectious and parasitic diseases	9,802	18.2	122	1.5	9,680	21.1	2,121	22.7	21.6	21.9
1. Tuberculosis	1,498	2.8	18	0.2	1,480	3.2	421	4.5	28.1	28.4
2. STDs excluding HIV	181	0.3	1	0.0	180	0.4	55	0.6	30.4	30.6
a. Syphilis	159	0.3	1	0.0	159	0.3	47	0.5	29.6	29.7
b. Chlamydia	13	0.0	0	0.0	13	0.0	5	0.1	38.7	38.8
c. Gonorrhea	8	0.0	0	0.0	8	0.0	3	0.0	33.9	33.9
d. Other STDs	1	0.0	0	0.0	0	0.0	0	0.0	0.0	0.0
3. HIV/AIDS	2,285	4.2	32	0.4	2,253	4.9	179	1.9	7.8	8.0
4. Diarrheal diseases	2,219	4.1	7	0.1	2,212	4.8	711	7.6	32.1	32.2
5. Childhood diseases	1,650	3.1	10	0.1	1,640	3.6	429	4.6	26.0	26.2
a. Pertussis	346	0.6	3	0.0	342	0.7	71	0.8	20.7	20.9

b. Poliomyelitis	2	0.0	0	0.0	2	0.0	1	0.0	29.7	29.7
c. Diphtheria	5	0.0	0	0.0	5	0.0	2	0.0	41.1	41.1
d. Measles	888	1.6	5	0.1	882	1.9	190	2.0	21.4	21.5
e. Tetanus	410	0.8	1	0.0	409	0.9	165	1.8	40.3	40.4
6. Meningitis	143	0.3	4	0.1	139	0.3	36	0.4	25.3	26.1
7. Hepatitis	92	0.2	4	0.1	88	0.2	16	0.2	17.0	17.7
8. Malaria	1,110	2.1	0	0.0	1,110	2.4	20	0.2	1.8	1.8
9. Tropical diseases	106	0.2	0	0.0	106	0.2	30	0.3	28.2	28.3
a. Trypanosomiasis	40	0.1	0	0.0	40	0.1	0	0.0	0.0	0.0
b. Chagas disease	17	0.0	0	0.0	17	0.0	0	0.0	0.0	0.0
c. Schistosomiasis	7	0.0	0	0.0	7	0.0	0	0.0	0.0	0.0
d. Leishmaniasis	42	0.1	0	0.0	42	0.1	30	0.3	70.8	70.9
e. lymphatic filariasis	0	0.0	0	0.0	0	0.0	0	0.0	::	:
f. Onchocerciasis	0	0.0	0	0.0	0	0.0	0	0.0	::	:
10. Leprosy	2	0.0	0	0.0	2	0.0	1	0.0	35.7	36.2
11. Dengue	15	0.0	0	0.0	15	0.0	10	0.1	63.2	63.2
12. Japanese encephalitis	3	0.0	0	0.0	3	0.0	1	0.0	23.3	23.3
13. Trachoma	0	0.0	0	0.0	0	0.0	0	0.0	0.0	..
14. Intestinal nematode infections	17	0.0	0	0.0	17	0.0	3	0.0	17.3	17.4
a. Ascariasis	8	0.0	0	0.0	8	0.0	1	0.0	14.2	14.2
b. Trichuriasis	5	0.0	0	0.0	5	0.0	0	0.0	9.3	9.3
c. Hookworm disease	4	0.0	0	0.0	4	0.0	1	0.0	35.0	35.0
d. Other intestinal infections	0	0.0	0	0.0	0	0.0	0	0.0	0.0	0.0
15. Other infectious diseases	478	0.9	46	0.6	432	0.9	209	2.2	43.7	48.4
B. Respiratory infections	3,507	6.5	309	3.9	3,198	7.0	987	10.6	28.1	30.9

(Table continues on the following page.)

Table 9A.2 (continued)

| CAUSE | WORLD | | HIGH-INCOME COUNTRIES | | LOW- AND MIDDLE-INCOME COUNTRIES | | INDIA TOTAL | | PERCENTAGE OF WORLD | PERCENTAGE LOW- AND MIDDLE-INCOME COUNTRIES |
	NUMBER (THOUSANDS)	PERCENT	NUMBER (THOUSANDS)	PERCENT	NUMBER (THOUSANDS)	PERCENT	NUMBER (THOUSANDS)	PERCENT		
1. Acute lower respiratory infections	3,452	6.4	306	3.8	3,146	6.9	969	10.4	28.1	30.8
2. Acute upper respiratory infections	34	0.1	3	0.0	31	0.1	10	0.1	28.3	31.0
3. Otitis media	20	0.0	0	0.0	20	0.0	9	0.1	42.1	42.6
C. Maternal conditions	493	0.9	2	0.0	491	1.1	125	1.3	25.3	25.4
1. Hemorrhage	123	0.2	0	0.0	122	0.3	30	0.3	24.4	24.5
2. Sepsis	74	0.1	0	0.0	74	0.2	20	0.2	26.9	27.0
3. Hypertensive disorders of pregnancy	62	0.1	1	0.0	61	0.1	15	0.2	24.3	24.5
4. Obstructed labor	38	0.1	0	0.0	38	0.1	10	0.1	26.6	26.7
5. Abortion	66	0.1	0	0.0	66	0.1	19	0.2	28.0	28.1
6. Other maternal conditions	131	0.2	0	0.0	130	0.3	31	0.3	24.0	24.0
D. Perinatal conditions	2,155	4.0	53	0.7	2,102	4.6	612	6.6	28.4	29.1
E. Nutritional deficiencies	490	0.9	23	0.3	467	1.0	100	1.1	20.4	21.4
1. Protein-energy malnutrition	281	0.5	7	0.1	274	0.6	53	0.6	19.0	19.5
2. Iodine deficiency	16	0.0	0	0.0	16	0.0	5	0.0	27.8	27.8

3. Vitamin A deficiency	78	0.1	0	0.0	78	0.2	16	0.2	20.2	20.2
4. Anemias	110	0.2	15	0.2	95	0.2	26	0.3	23.6	27.4
5. Other nutritional disorders	4	0.0	1	0.0	3	0.0	0	0.0	0.0	0.0
II. Noncommunicable conditions	31,717	58.8	7,024	87.4	24,693	53.8	4,470	47.9	14.1	18.1
A. Malignant neoplasms	7,228	13.4	2,020	25.1	5,209	11.3	653	7.0	9.0	12.5
1. Mouth and oropharynx	352	0.7	41	0.5	312	0.7	100	1.1	28.4	32.1
2. Esophagus	436	0.8	49	0.6	387	0.8	62	0.7	14.3	16.1
3. Stomach	822	1.5	143	1.8	679	1.5	51	0.5	6.2	7.5
4. Colon/rectum	556	1.0	243	3.0	313	0.7	25	0.3	4.5	8.1
5. Liver	609	1.1	46	0.6	563	1.2	16	0.2	2.6	2.8
6. Pancreas	214	0.4	99	1.2	115	0.3	9	0.1	4.3	8.0
7. Trachea/bronchus/lung	1,244	2.3	422	5.3	822	1.8	79	0.8	6.3	9.6
8. Melanoma and other skin cancers	55	0.1	25	0.3	30	0.1	1	0.0	2.4	4.4
9. Breast	412	0.8	160	2.0	252	0.5	47	0.5	11.4	18.6
10. Cervix	237	0.4	17	0.2	220	0.5	57	0.6	24.2	26.1
11. Corpus uteri	73	0.1	27	0.3	46	0.1	4	0.0	5.7	9.1
12. Ovary	122	0.2	45	0.6	76	0.2	14	0.2	11.7	18.6
13. Prostate	239	0.4	115	1.4	124	0.3	14	0.1	5.9	11.3
14. Bladder	158	0.3	56	0.7	101	0.2	8	0.1	5.3	8.3
15. Lymphoma	248	0.5	91	1.1	157	0.3	22	0.2	8.9	14.0
16. Leukaemia	253	0.5	65	0.8	188	0.4	18	0.2	7.3	9.8
17. Other cancers	1,199	2.2	373	4.6	825	1.8	124	1.3	10.4	15.1
B. Other neoplasms	109	0.2	39	0.5	69	0.2	5	0.1	4.6	7.2
C. Diabetes mellitus	600	1.1	161	2.0	439	1.0	102	1.1	17.0	23.2

(Table continues on the following page.)

311

Table 9A.2 (continued)

CAUSE	WORLD NUMBER (THOUSANDS)	WORLD PERCENT	HIGH-INCOME COUNTRIES NUMBER (THOUSANDS)	HIGH-INCOME COUNTRIES PERCENT	LOW- AND MIDDLE-INCOME COUNTRIES NUMBER (THOUSANDS)	LOW- AND MIDDLE-INCOME COUNTRIES PERCENT	INDIA TOTAL NUMBER (THOUSANDS)	INDIA TOTAL PERCENT	INDIA PERCENTAGE OF WORLD	INDIA PERCENTAGE LOW- AND MIDDLE-INCOME COUNTRIES
D. Nutritional/endocrine disorders	147	0.3	50	0.6	96	0.2	2	0.0	1.4	2.1
E. Neuropsychiatric disorders	720	1.3	225	2.8	495	1.1	104	1.1	14.4	21.0
1. Unipolar major depression	0	0.0	0	0.0	0	0.0	0	0.0	..	..
2. Bipolar affective disorder	16	0.0	1	0.0	15	0.0	2	0.0	15.7	16.3
3. Psychoses	54	0.1	14	0.2	40	0.1	5	0.1	8.7	11.8
4. Epilepsy	68	0.1	8	0.1	60	0.1	13	0.1	18.8	21.2
5. Alcohol dependence	59	0.1	16	0.2	42	0.1	5	0.1	9.0	12.5
6. Alzheimer and other dementias	216	0.4	105	1.3	111	0.2	22	0.2	10.1	19.5
7. Parkinson's disease	63	0.1	33	0.4	30	0.1	6	0.1	9.8	20.9
8. Multiple sclerosis	26	0.0	6	0.1	20	0.0	3	0.0	12.5	16.1
9. Drug dependence	11	0.0	3	0.0	7	0.0	0	0.0	2.3	3.4
10. Post traumatic stress disorder	0	0.0	0	0.0	0	0.0	0	0.0	..	..
11. Obsessive-compulsive disorders	0	0.0	0	0.0	0	0.0	0	0.0	..	..
12. Panic disorders	0	0.0	0	0.0	0	0.0	0	0.0	..	..
13. Other neuropsychiatric disorders	208	0.4	38	0.5	170	0.4	47	0.5	22.7	27.8

Cause										
F. Sense organ disorders	20	0.0	0	0.0	20	0.0	0	0.0	0.2	0.2
1. Glaucoma	6	0.0	0	0.0	6	0.0	0	0.0	0.0	0.0
2. Cataracts	6	0.0	0	0.0	6	0.0	0	0.0	0.0	0.0
3. Other sense organ disorders	7	0.0	0	0.0	7	0.0	0	0.0	0.5	0.5
G. Cardiovascular diseases	16,690	30.9	3,592	44.7	13,098	28.5	2,820	30.2	16.9	21.5
1. Rheumatic heart disease	383	0.7	22	0.3	361	0.8	86	0.9	22.4	23.7
2. Ischemic heart disease	7,375	13.7	1,884	23.5	5,492	12.0	1,471	15.8	19.9	26.8
3. Cerebrovascular disease	5,106	9.5	893	11.1	4,213	9.2	557	6.0	10.9	13.2
4. Inflammatory cardiac disease	548	1.0	74	0.9	474	1.0	100	1.1	18.2	21.1
5. Other cardiac diseases	3,277	6.1	719	9.0	2,558	5.6	606	6.5	18.5	23.7
H. Respiratory diseases	2,995	5.6	391	4.9	2,604	5.7	284	3.0	9.5	10.9
1. Chronic obstructive pulmonary disease	2,249	4.2	280	3.5	1,969	4.3	153	1.6	6.8	7.7
2. Asthma	144	0.3	24	0.3	120	0.3	21	0.2	14.8	17.7
3. Other respiratory diseases	602	1.1	87	1.1	515	1.1	110	1.2	18.2	21.3
I. Digestive diseases	1,783	3.3	322	4.0	1,461	3.2	240	2.6	13.4	16.4
1. Peptic ulcer disease	174	0.3	33	0.4	141	0.3	41	0.4	23.4	28.9
2. Cirrhosis of the liver	775	1.4	122	1.5	653	1.4	144	1.5	18.6	22.1
3. Appendicitis	48	0.1	2	0.0	47	0.1	11	0.1	22.3	23.0
4. Other digestive diseases	786	1.5	165	2.1	621	1.4	44	0.5	5.6	7.1

(Table continues on the following page.)

Table 9A.2 (continued)

CAUSE	WORLD		HIGH-INCOME COUNTRIES		LOW- AND MIDDLE-INCOME COUNTRIES		INDIA TOTAL		PERCENTAGE OF WORLD	PERCENTAGE LOW- AND MIDDLE-INCOME COUNTRIES
	NUMBER (THOUSANDS)	PERCENT	NUMBER (THOUSANDS)	PERCENT	NUMBER (THOUSANDS)	PERCENT	NUMBER (THOUSANDS)	PERCENT		
J. Diseases of the genito-urinary system	765	1.4	139	1.7	626	1.4	102	1.1	13.4	16.3
1. Nephritis/nephrosis	554	1.0	90	1.1	464	1.0	89	1.0	16.1	19.3
2. Benign prostatic hypertrophy	33	0.1	4	0.1	29	0.1	11	0.1	31.9	36.7
3. Other genito-urinary system diseases	178	0.3	45	0.6	133	0.3	2	0.0	1.3	1.7
K. Skin diseases	44	0.1	13	0.2	30	0.1	2	0.0	5.4	7.7
L. Musculoskeletal diseases	100	0.2	35	0.4	65	0.1	3	0.0	2.5	3.8
1. Rheumatoid arthritis	17	0.0	10	0.1	7	0.0	2	0.0	10.6	25.9
2. Osteoarthritis	0	0.0	0	0.0	0	0.0	0	0.0	0.0	0.0
3. Other musculo-skeletal diseases	83	0.2	25	0.3	58	0.1	1	0.0	0.9	1.2
M. Congenital abnormalities	515	1.0	36	0.5	478	1.0	153	1.6	29.8	32.1
N. Oral diseases	2	0.0	0	0.0	2	0.0	0	0.0	18.7	23.0
1. Dental caries	0	0.0	0	0.0	0	0.0	0	0.0	..	..
2. Periodontal disease	0	0.0	0	0.0	0	0.0	0	0.0	0.0	0.0
3. Edentulism	0	0.0	0	0.0	0	0.0	0	0.0	..	..
4. Other oral diseases	2	0.0	0	0.0	2	0.0	0	0.0	18.8	23.0

III. Injuries	5,765	10.7	498	6.2	5,266	11.5	923	9.9	16.0	17.5
A. Unintentional	3,493	6.5	327	4.1	3,166	6.9	723	7.7	20.7	22.8
1. Road traffic accidents	1,171	2.2	142	1.8	1,029	2.2	217	2.3	18.5	21.1
2. Poisoning	252	0.5	14	0.2	238	0.5	32	0.3	12.5	13.3
3. Falls	316	0.6	77	1.0	239	0.5	50	0.5	15.9	21.0
4. Fires	282	0.5	11	0.1	271	0.6	135	1.4	47.7	49.6
5. Drowning	495	0.9	13	0.2	482	1.1	92	1.0	18.5	19.0
6. Other unintentional injuries	977	1.8	70	0.9	907	2.0	199	2.1	20.3	21.9
B. Intentional	2,272	4.2	172	2.1	2,100	4.6	200	2.1	8.8	9.5
1. Self-inflicted	948	1.8	130	1.6	818	1.8	124	1.3	13.1	15.2
2. Homicide and violence	736	1.4	38	0.5	698	1.5	72	0.8	9.8	10.3
3. War	588	1.1	4	0.0	584	1.3	4	0.0	0.6	0.6

.. Negligible.
Note: STD, sexually transmitted disease.
Source: WHO (1999).

Table 9A.3 Comparison of India and Other Countries on Selected Health-Related Indicators, Selected Years, 1992–99

COUNTRY	POPULATION, 1999 (MILLIONS)	GNP PER CAPITA, 1999 (U.S. DOLLARS)	POPULATION BELOW US$1 PER DAY, 1992-98 (PERCENT)	ILLITERATE ADULT FEMALES, 1998 (PERCENT)	LIFE EXPECTANCY, 1999 (DISABILITY-ADJUSTED LIFE YEARS)	INFANT MORTALITY, 1998 (PER 1,000 POPULATION)	TOTAL FERTILITY RATE, 1998 (LIFETIME BIRTHS PER WOMAN AGES 15 TO 49)	MALNUTRITION OF CHILDREN UNDER AGE 5, 1992-98 (PERCENT)[a]
India	998	450	44.2	57	53.2	72	3.3	53[a]
Low-income countries	2,417	410	36.0	49		68	3.1	36
Nigeria	124	310	70.2	48	38.3	76	5.3	39
Bangladesh	128	370	29.1	71	49.9	73	3.1	56
Pakistan	135	470	31.0	71	55.9	91	4.9	38
Indonesia	207	580	15.2	20	59.7	43	2.7	34
Middle-income countries	2,667	2,000	8.2	20		31	2.5	12
China	1,250	780	18.5	25	62.3	31	1.9	16
Sri Lanka	19	820	6.6	12	62.8	16	2.1	38
South Africa	42	3,160	11.5	16	39.8	51	2.8	9
Brazil	168	4,420	5.1	16	59.1	33	2.3	6
High-income countries	891	27,730	0.1	..		6	1.7	..
United Kingdom	59	22,640		..	71.7	6	1.7	..
United States	273	30,600		..	70.0	7	2.0	1
World	5,975	4,890	24.0	32		54	2.7	30

.. Negligible.

Note: Blank spaces denote that calculations have not been done on regional disability-adjusted life expectancy.

a. Weight more than 2 standard deviations below average for age; in 1999, proportion of children under age 3 who fit this definition was 47 percent.

Source: World Bank (2000d); WHO (2000c).

Table 9A.4 Causes of DALYs Lost in India, 1990 and 1998

CAUSE	DEATHS PER 1,000 POPULATION			PROPORTION OF DEATHS (PERCENT)			DALYs LOST PER 1,000 POPULATION		PROPORTION OF DALYs LOST (PERCENT)	
	1990	1998	CHANGE (PERCENT)	1990	1998	CHANGE	1990	1998	1990	1998
Communicable diseases, maternal and perinatal conditions, and nutritional deficiencies	5.6	4.0	−28.6	51.0	42.2	−17.3	191.0	137.7	56.4	50.3
Noncommunicable conditions	4.5	4.6	2.2	40.4	47.9	18.6	98.2	90.3	29.0	33.0
Injuries	1.0	0.9	−10.0	8.6	9.9	15.1	49.3	45.8	14.6	16.7
Total	11.0	9.5	−13.6	100.0	100.0	0	338.5	273.8	100.0	100.0

Note: DALY, disability-adjusted life year.
Source: Murray and Lopez (1996); WHO (2000c).

Table 9A.5 Infant Mortality and Total Fertility Rates in India and Major Indian States, 1981–97

STATE	POPULATION, 1999 (MILLIONS)	INFANT MORTALITY RATE, 1998 (PER 1,000 LIVE BIRTHS)	REDUCTION IN RURAL IMR, 1981–97 (PERCENT)	TOTAL FERTILITY RATE, 1997	REDUCTION IN RURAL TFR, 1981–97 (PERCENT)
India	981.3	72	34	3.3	24.5
Group A: *TFR of 2.1 or less*					
Kerala	32.0	16	64	1.8	37.9
Tamil Nadu	61.3	53	40	2.0	40.5
Group B: *TFR of more than 2.1 and less than 3.0*					
Karnataka	51.4	58	14	2.5	35.7
Andhra Pradesh	74.6	66	17	2.5	28.2
West Bengal	78.0	53	38	2.6	28.6
Maharashtra	90.1	49	30	2.7	37.5
Punjab	23.3	54	35	2.7	22.0
Group C: *TFR of at least 3.0*					
Orissa	35.5	98	26	3.0	28.3
Gujarat	47.6	64	44	3.0	25.0
Assam	25.6	78	47	3.2	19.0
Haryana	19.5	69	31	3.4	26.9
Madhya Pradesh	78.3	98	29	4.0	20.0
Rajasthan	52.6	83	25	4.2	23.7
Bihar	98.1	67	36	4.4	20.7
Uttar Pradesh	166.4	85	44	4.8	16.4

Note: IMR, infant mortality rate; TFR, total fertility rate. Within groups, states are listed in order of TFR. IMR refers to infants less than 1 year of age; TFR is lifetime births per woman ages 15–49. Major Indian states are those with a population of more than 15 million. Bihar includes Jharkhand, Madhya Pradesh includes Chatisgarh, and Uttar Pradesh includes Uttaranchal.
Source: Registrar General (2000).

Table 9A.6 Underweight Children under Three Years of Age in Major States of India, 1998–99
(percent)

STATE	PERCENT
Madhya Pradesh	55
Bihar	54
Orissa	54
Uttar Pradesh	52
Rajasthan	51
Maharashtra	50
West Bengal	49
Gujarat	45
Karnataka	44
Andhra Pradesh	38
Tamil Nadu	37
Assam	36
Haryana	35
Punjab	29
Kerala	27

Note: Underweight children are those whose weights are statistically low for their ages (that is, more than 2 standard deviations below average). Major Indian states are those with populations of more than 15 million. Bihar includes Jharkhand, Madhya Pradesh includes Chatisgarh, and Uttar Pradesh includes Uttaranchal.
Source: IIPS (2000).

Table 9A.7 Reduction in Rates of Severe and Total Malnutrition (Weight for Age) among Children in India and Major States in India between 1992–93 and 1998–99

(percent)

AREA	SEVERE	TOTAL
India	6.40	2.60
Andhra Pradesh	11.40	5.30
Assam	14.40	5.40
Bihar	8.20	5.60
Gujarat	5.00	1.40
Haryana	3.30	–1.10
Karnataka	10.40	2.90
Kerala	1.60	1.40
Madhya Pradesh	2.30	–2.00
Maharashtra	4.60	3.70
Orissa	–1.10	2.00
Punjab	17.20	5.40
Rajasthan	–9.00	–1.60
Tamil Nadu	11.50	2.70
Uttar Pradesh	7.30	2.70
West Bengal	8.10	2.10

Note: Negative values denote an increase. Malnutrition in 1992–93 was measured among children under age 4; in 1998–99, under age 3. Severe malnutrition is weight more than 2 standard deviations below average for age; total malnutrition is weight more than 3 standard deviations below average. Major Indian states are those with populations of more than 15 million. Bihar includes Jharkhand, Madhya Pradesh includes Chatisgarh, and Uttar Pradesh includes Uttaranchal.
Source: IIPS (2000).

Table 9A.8 Comparison of Female and Male Health Outcomes in India, 1998–99

SEX AND RATIO	MORTALITY PER 1,000 LIVE BIRTHSᵃ				INDICATORS FOR CHILDREN UNDER AGE 3ᵇ			TUBERCULOSIS UNDER MEDICAL TREATMENT (PER 100,000 POPULATION)
	NEO-NATAL	POST-NEO-NATAL	INFANT	UNDER 5	UNDER-WEIGHT (PERCENT)	ACUTE RESPIRATORY INFECTION IN PAST 2 WEEKS (PERCENT)	DIARRHEA IN PAST 2 WEEKS (PERCENT)	
Female	44.6	26.6	71.1	105.2	48.9	17.9	18.9	357
Male	50.7	24.2	74.8	97.9	45.3	20.7	19.4	502
Female-male ratio	0.88	1.10	0.95	1.07	1.08	0.86	0.97	0.71

a. Mortality rates are for the 10-year period preceding the survey. Neonatal denotes birth to less than one month of age; post-neonatal, one month to less than one year; infant, birth to one year; under five, birth to under five.
b. Underweight is weight that is more than 2 standard deviations below average for age.
Source: IIPS (2000).

Notes

1.   The Census of India 2001 provisional population estimates report sex ratios of between 927 and 934 in each of the four censuses between 1971 and 2001 (table 10 of the results posted at www.censusindia.net/ on April 26, 2001).

2.   The states are Bihar, Jharkhand, Uttar Pradesh, West Bengal, Orissa, Madhya Pradesh, and Chatisgarh.

3.   Private health spending as a proportion of total expenditure is distributed more progressively. For example, the richest quintile spends 6.6 percent of its total expenditure on health, compared with 3.8 percent for the poorest quintile.

4.   Estimates of the true effect of hospitalization on poverty levels may require more intensive studies involving prospective analysis of hospitalization, income, and consumption.

5. We assumed conservatively that all the money borrowed for hospitalization would not have been spent if people were not ill. Including borrowing raises the level to 35 percent.

6. An additional 3.3 percent of hospitalized Indians fall below the poverty line if indirect medical expenses, such as transport costs, are also included.

7. The definitions and methodologies for this area of inquiry are the least developed of the three health system outcomes and are least amenable to international or interstate comparisons. We use a different definition of responsiveness than does the World Health Organization's *World Health Report 2000*, which refers to the non-medical aspects of care and excludes satisfaction; in contrast, we look specifically at satisfaction and the legal protection of the public from negligence and redress.

8. Equal access to health care is listed under the Directive Principles of the Constitution, but not explicitly as a fundamental right. The courts, however, have held that the fundamental right to life includes health care (Background Paper 9).

9. More detailed analysis and specific recommendations for improving patient redress are provided in Background Paper 10.

10. The alternative hypothesis—that people are receiving high quality medical care and therefore do not complain—is highly unlikely, according to reviewers of quality of the private sector (Background Papers 6–8).

11. The study used an adapted and translated version of a 51-item patient satisfaction questionnaire.

12. This study used an adapted and translated version of an 11-item visit satisfaction questionnaire.

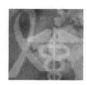

APPENDIX A

Studies Conducted for the Present Report

STUDY	RESEARCH ORGANIZATION	POLICY QUESTIONS ADDRESSED	USE OF STUDY RESULTS
1. Private Health Sector Market Analysis a. Systematic Review of Knowledge b. Field Analysis in Andhra Pradesh (AP) and Uttar Pradesh (UP)	a. Indian Institute of Technology; Center for Enquiry into Health and Allied Themes (CEHAT); Jawaharlal Nehru University (funded by WHO) b. Institute of Health Systems (AP); Indian Institute of Management—Lucknow (UP)	How can India take advantage of the private sector to meet social goals?	• Better understanding of constraints, incentives, and subsidies and of how the private sector functions are to influence policy proposals and project design • New partnerships in service delivery and financing of health services • New approaches to regulation and quality assurance • New public accountabilities • Benchmarks for standards
2. Consumer Protection in Health: Legal Framework and Current Practices a. Legal framework for health b. Mechanisms of consumer redress	a. Indian Law Institute b. Voluntary Organization in Interest of Consumer Education	How can consumers become more empowered over health issues?	• Better understanding of role of consumer laws • Better public advocacy
3. Health Financing Options: Health Insurance a. Critical analysis of Indian experience b. Prospect of insurance and regulation in India c. Effects of private health insurance on the poor and the health system—international experience	a. Institute of Economic Growth b. National Council for Applied Economic Research c. Fereirro (Chile)	How can health insurance be used to improve equity and efficiency of health services and how can India minimize the negative effects of health insurance liberalization?	• Insurance regulations to minimize harm to poor • Increased capacity of technical staff to deal with insurance issues • New experiments with health insurance for the poor

4. Pharmaceuticals Analysis a. Pharmaceuticals sector analysis in three states b. Pharmaceuticals industry analysis	a. Benaras Hindu University (UP); Kilpak Medical College (Tamil Nadu); JSS College of Pharmacy (Karnataka); IHBAS (Delhi); b. Administrative Staff College of India (AP)	How can safe, effective, affordable drugs be accessible to Indians, whether through the private or public sector?	• Revise design of new projects and improvement of supervision of pharmaceuticals lending • Revised drug policies; new efforts on quality assurance and regulation of private sector • Preparation for TRIPS
5. Quality of Health Services	National Quality Assurance Council formed from eminent physicians. Subpanel work convened by AIIMS, CEHAT, HAP, MGRMU.	How can India systematically improve quality assurance in health at national and state levels?	• New institutions and networks for quality assurance • New modalities and systems for quality assurance • Hospital accreditation scheme
6. Distribution of Health Benefits and Costs	National Council on Applied Economic Research (with NIPFP and IEG)	How well do public and private health services reach the poor?	Better problem identification, monitoring, and advocacy to ensure the focus of HNP efforts is on the poor
7. Critical Issues in Decentralizing Health Responsibilities (DFID funding)	National Institute of Rural Development—Hyderabad	How can India best reorganize its programs around districts and local bodies?	• Identification of how to strengthen capacity of states and PRIs in health sector • Options for streamlining and integrating health programs
8. Options for Reorganizing Public Hospitals (DFID funding)	Institute for Health Systems Development (U.K.) plus local counterparts	How can hospitals and health facilities be reorganized to become more efficient, equitable?	New experiments in hospital organization

Note: WHO, World Health Organization; JSS, Jagadguru Sri Shivarathreeshwara; IHBAS, Institute of Human Behavior and Allied Sciences; TRIPS, trade-related aspects of intellectual property; AIIMS, All Indian Institute of Medical Sciences; HAP, Health Action for People; MGRMU, The Tamil Nadu Dr. M. G. R. Medical University; NIPFP, National Institute of Public Finance and Policy; IEG, Institute of Economic Growth; HNP, Health, Nutrition and Population (The World Bank); DFID, Department for International Development; PRI, Panchayati Raj Institutions.

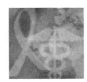

Background Papers

These papers, prepared in support of the present report, are available on the web site of the World Bank, at http://wbln0018.worldbank.org/SAR/India/HealthESW/AR/cover. nsf/HomePage/1?OpenDocument

1. Garg, C. "Implications of Current Experiences in Health Insurance in India."

2. Mahal, A. "Private Entry into Health Insurance in India: An Assessment."

3. Ferreiro, A. "Private Health Insurance in India: Would Its Implementation Affect the Poor?"

4. Nandraj, S. "Accreditation System for Hospitals in India."

5. Mahal, A., J. Singh, F. Afridi, V. Lamba, A. Gumber, and V. Selvaraju. "Who 'Benefits' from Public Sector Health Spending in India? Results of a Benefit Incidence Analysis for India."

6. Nandraj, S. "Contracting and Regulation in the Health Sector: Concerns, Challenges, and Options."

7. Muraleedharan, V.R. "Private-Public Partnership in Health Care Sector in India: A Review of Policy Options and Challenges."

8. Baru, R.V., I. Qadeer, and R. Priya. "Critical Review of Studies on the Private Sector in Health."

9. Indian Law Institute. "Legal Framework for Health Care in India: Experience and Future Directions."

10. Misra, B., and P. Kalra. "The Regulatory Framework for Consumer Redress in the Healthcare System in India."

11. Pearson, M. "International Experience of Hospital Autonomy."

12. Pearson, M. "Overview Paper: Hospital Autonomy in India."

13. Administrative Staff College of India. "The Indian Pharmaceuticals Industry."

14. Govindaraj, R., and G. Chellaraj. "Pharmaceuticals Sector in India: Issues and Options."

15. Kilpauk Medical College, Department of Community Medicine. "Pharmaceutical Study on Drug Policy: Tamil Nadu."

16. Benaras Hindu University. "Drug Policy Assessment Study: Uttar Pradesh."

17. JSS College of Pharmacy. "Drug Policy Assessment Study: Karnataka."

18. Mahal, A., A. Yazbeck, D.H. Peters, and G.N.V. Ramana, "The Poor and Health Service Use in India."

19. Peters, D.H., A. Yazbeck, G.N.V. Ramana, and R. Sharma. "Public-Private Partnerships in Health, Background Paper: Issues and Options."

20. Institute of Health Systems. "Private Health Sector Market Analysis in Andhra Pradesh."

21. Indian Institute of Management—Lucknow. "Private Health Sector Market Analysis in Uttar Pradesh."

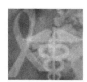

Major Recommendations of National Health Policy Reports since Independence

Bhore Committee, 1946

- No individual should lack access to medical care because of inability to pay for it.
- Special emphasis should be placed on preventive methods and on communicable diseases.
- Health services should be as "close to the people as possible in order to ensure the maximum benefit to the community to be served."
- All facilities for diagnosis and treatment should be available in the public health services when it is fully developed.
- One primary health unit per 10,000-20,000 population with 75 beds, 6 doctors, and 6 public health nurses
- One bed per 175 population; one doctor per 1,600 population and one nurse per 600 population
- One 650-bed hospital at taluka level (300,000 population) and one district hospital of 2,500 beds
- No patents in pharmaceutical products
- 15 percent of government expenditure to be devoted to health care.

Mudaliar Committee, 1961

- Strengthen primary health centers (PHCs)
- One PHC per 40,000 population that lacks hospital services
- One bed per 1,000 population and one doctor per 3,000 population
- One 50-bed basic specialty hospital for each taluka and one 500-bed district hospital
- Central government to control communicable diseases
- One medical college per 5 million population
- Only process patents for 5–10 years for drugs
- No integration of systems of medicine

Jain Committee, 1966

- One bed per 1,000 population
- One 50-bed hospital at taluka level
- Enhance maternity facilities at each level
- Health insurance for a larger population coverage
- Charge for health access to augment resources

Kartar Singh Committee, 1974

- Integration of all health programs and health workers: retrain health workers as multipurpose workers
- A team of one male and one female worker at subcenter level (3,000 population)
- One PHC per 50,000 population
- One health supervisor for every four health workers

Srivastava Committee, 1975

- One male and one female health worker per 5,000 population
- One health assistant per two health workers
- One additional doctor and nurse at PHC for maternal and child health services

- Increase PHC drug budgets
- Compulsory national service of two years at PHC by every doctor between fifth and fifteenth year of career
- Establish medical and health education commission
- Integration of various health systems

Indian Council for Medical Research–Indian Council for Social Science Research Joint Panel, 1980

- A village health unit per 1,000 population with one male and one female health worker
- One subcenter per 5,000 population with one male and one female health worker
- One 30-bed community health center per 100,000 population with 6 general doctors and 3 specialists
- A district health center for every 1 million population and a specialist center for every 5 million population
- No further expansion of medical education and drug production but only their rationalization and reorientation
- 6 percent of GNP must be ultimately spent on health care services

National Health Policy, 1983

- Provision of universal, comprehensive primary health care services
- Involvement of private practitioners and NGOs to expand coverage of and access to services
- Train village-based workers in simple skills
- Evolve a decentralized system of health care and establish a referral systems
- Establish a nationwide chain of epidemiological stations
- Encourage private investment in health sector to reduce government burden
- Selected health and demographic targets to be achieved by 2000

National Population Policy, 2000

- Seek a mix of sociodemographic and health goals for 2010 with the primary aim of bringing the total fertility rate to replacement level
- Increase outreach and coverage of comprehensive package of reproductive and child health services by government in partnership with NGOs and the private sector
- Create one-stop, integrated service delivery at the village level
- Expand public health infrastructure by increasing numbers of subcenters, primary health centers, and community health centers
- Decentralize planning and program implementation with high involvement of the Panchayati Raj Institutions (PRIs) and community groups
- Promote intersectoral approach among key government departments
- Establish a national commission on population with equivalent structures at the state level
- Set up a National Technical Committee with medical experts and government representatives
- Double the annual budget of the Family Welfare Department
- Create incentives to promote the small-family norm

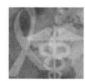

APPENDIX D

Efforts to Address the Role of Private Providers in National Tuberculosis Control Programs

LOCATION	PRACTICES
Congo, Dem. Rep. of	National Tuberculosis Control Programs (NTP) provide team training to a doctor, a laboratory technician, and a nurse from Kinshasa city hospitals and polyclinics. Drugs are subsidized. Patients are managed according to guidelines.
Egypt, Arab Rep. of	Prominent private chest physicians on NTP board. Pilot projects are started with five university hospitals adopting directly observed treatment short-course (DOTS). Continuing tuberculosis (TB) education for in-practice chest physicians initiated; modifications to TB education in medical curricula planned. In another pilot, private laboratories report results of all sputum tests to the NTP.
India	A few running and evolving models: • A private nonprofit hospital runs a DOTS project for patients referred by private general practitioners; DOT done in neighborhood centers located in private nursing homes, clinics, and private and nongovernmental organization dispensaries. • A voluntary organization acts as an interface between private providers and NTP to facilitate referrals; and DOT by private providers. • NTP treatment supervisors assign diagnosed patients to their preferred private practitioner agreeing to do DOTS, maintain records, and report default. • Local association of doctors tries out graded involvement of private providers ranging from referral to running a DOTS program.

Kenya	Anti-TB Association provides subsidized drugs to private hospitals and chest physicians in Nairobi who in turn follow NTP guidelines, notify cases, assist in defaulter retrieval, and maintain and submit records.
Morocco	Two successive yearly surveys show good TB management practices of private practitioners. Forty percent of patients referred to NTP are from private sector. Probable reasons for good management practices of private doctors: undergraduate medical curricula provide substantial time for training in TB, and all postgraduates have to work within NTP before getting license to practice.
New York, New York, United States	Upgrading and improving the clinical services offered by chest clinics located throughout the city. State-of-the-art and confidential services including DOTS provided free of cost to suspects and patients, including treatment for latent infection to high-risk individuals, social services, and HIV counseling and testing. Result: a four-fold increase in referrals from private sector. Obligatory for laboratories to report results of sputum smears and those of drug susceptibility testing.
Korea, Rep. of	NTP surveys private providers' TB management practices and treatment outcomes and shares results with the providers. Improved performance demonstrated in a subsequent survey.
Syrian Arab Rep.	Dissatisfied by private physicians' poor response to persistent and varied approaches to involve them, the NTP manager persuaded the Minister of Health to ban sale of anti-TB drugs in private pharmacies. Effectiveness yet to be evaluated.
Netherlands	Involvement of private providers at all levels including representation on TB Control Policy Committee. Clarity and consensus on roles to be played by the public and private sectors in managing each patient.
Philippines	NTP supports two projects: a university hospital and an expensive private hospital in Manila, which run effective DOTS clinics.

Note: NTP, National Tuberculosis Control Programs; DOTS, directly observed treatment short-course; TB, tuberculosis.
Source: WHO (2001).

Bibliography

The set of 21 background papers prepared in support of the present report are listed in appendix B.

The word *processed* describes informally reproduced works that may not be commonly available through libraries.

Administrative Staff College of India. 1995. "Beneficiary Assessment for the Karnataka State Health Systems Development Project." Processed.

Antia, N. H. n.d. "Voluntary Organizations and Health Care in India." Foundation for Research in Community Health, Mumbai.

Arrow, Kenneth J. 1963. "Uncertainty and the Welfare Economics of Medical Care. *American Economic Review* 53:941–69.

Ashtekar, S., and D. Mankad. 2001. "Who Cares? Rural Health Practitioners in Maharashtra." *Economic and Political Weekly*, February 3-10, 448–53.

BAIF (Bharatiya Agro Industries Foundation). 1997. "Traditional Medicine in Rural Tribal Areas in India." BAIF Development Research Foundation, Pune, Maharashtra.

Bajaj, J. S. 1996. "Report of the Expert Committee on Public Health System." Ministry of Health and Family Welfare, New Delhi.

Balambal, R., K. Faggarajamma, and F. Rahman. 1997. "Impact of Tuberculosis on Private For-Profit Providers." Tuberculosis Research Centre, Chennai, Tamil Nadu. Processed.

Barr, N. 1990. "Economic Theory and the Welfare State: A Survey and Reinterpretation. Welfare State Programme." Discussion Paper No. 54. London School of Economics and Political Science, London.

Baru, R. V. 1998. *Private Health Care in India: Social Characteristics and Trends.* New Delhi: Sage Publications.

Basu, S. 2000. "Policy for the Reform of the Drug Control Authority: A Stakeholder Analysis." Processed.

Bennett, S., and V. R. Muraleedharan. 2000. "'New Public Management' and Health Care in Third World." *Economic and Political Weekly,* January 8, 59–68.

Berman, P. 1995. "Health Sector Reform: Making Health Development Sustainable." In P. Berman, ed., *Health Sector Reform in Developing Countries.* Boston: Harvard School of Public Health.

———. 1996. "Health Care Expenditure in India." In M. Das Gupta, L. Chen, and T. N. Krishnan, eds., *Health, Poverty and Development in India.* New Delhi: Oxford University Press.

———. 2000. "Organization of Ambulatory Care Provision: A Critical Determinant of Health System Performance in Developing Countries. *Bulletin of the World Health Organization* 78:791–802.

Berman, P., and M. E. Khan, eds. 1993. *Paying for India's Health Care.* New Delhi: Sage Publications.

Bhandari, N. 1992. "The Household Management of Diarrhoea in the Social Context: A Study of a Delhi Slum." Ph.D. diss. Jawaharlal Nehru University, New Delhi.

Bhat, P. N. 1995. "Maternal Mortality in India: Estimates from Regression Model." *Studies in Family Planning* 26:217–32.

Bhat, R. 1996a. "Regulating the Private Health Care Sector: The Case of the Indian Consumer Protection Act." *Health Policy and Planning* 11:265–79.

———. 1996b. "Regulation of the Private Health Sector in India." *International Journal of Health Planning and Management* 11:253–74.

Bhore, J., R. A. Amesur, and A. C. Banerjee. 1946. *Report of the Health Survey and Development Committee.* Vol. I. Government of India, New Delhi.

Blackstone Ltd. 2000. "West Bengal Health Systems Development Project: Quality Assurance Programme." Draft Report. Processed.

Cai, W. W., J. S. Marks, C. H. Chen, Y. X. Zhuang, L. Morris, and J. R. Harris. 1998. "Increased Cesarean Section Rates and Emerging Patterns of Health Insurance in Shanghai, China." *American Journal of Public Health* 88:777–80.

Caldwell, J. C., and G. Santow. 1989. "Introduction." In J. C. Caldwell and G. Santow, eds., *Selected Readings in The Cultural, Social, and Behavioural Determinants of Health*. Canberra: The Australian National University.

Cassels, A. 1995. "Health Sector Reform: Key Issues in Less Developed Countries. *Journal of International Health Development* 7:329–49.

CBHI (Central Bureau of Health Intelligence). Various years. *Health Information of India*. Annual. Ministry of Health and Family Welfare, Directorate General of Health Services. New Delhi.

Census Commissioner of India. 1981. *Census of India*. Ministry of Home Affairs. New Delhi.

Centre for Policy Research. 1999. *Report on the Restructuring the Ministry of Health & Family Welfare*. New Delhi.

Chaix-Couturier, C., I. Durand-Zaleski, D. Jolly, and P. Durieux. 2000. "Effects of Financial Incentives on Medical Practice: Results from a Systematic Review of the Literature and Methodological Issues. *International Journal for Quality in Health Care* 12:133–42.

Chand, S. K. 1988. "The Traditional Herbal Medicine System of Chotanagpur: A Study of Its Present Status and Future Prospects." Xavier Institute of Social Service, Ranchi, Jharkhand. Processed.

Chawla, M. 2000. "Private and Pubic Markets for Physician Services in Developing Countries: Evidence of Inter-Linkages." Processed.

Chollet, D. J., and M. Lewis. 1997. "Private Insurance: Principles and Practice." In G. Schieber, ed., *Innovations in Health Care Financing*. Proceedings of a World Bank Conference, March 10–11, 1997. World Bank Discussion Paper 365. Washington, D.C.

Claeson, M., E. R. Bos, and I. Pathamanathan. 1999. *Reducing Child Mortality in India: Keeping Up the Pace*. Washington, D.C: World Bank.

De Regt, R., H. L. Minkoff, J. Feldman, and R. H. Schwarz. 1986. "Relation of Private or Clinic Care to the Cesarean Birth Rate." *New England Journal of Medicine* 315:619–24.

Dohrenwend, B., and B. Dohrenwend. 1969. *Social Status and Psychological Disorder: A Causal Inquiry*. New York: John Wiley and Sons.

Dreze, J., and A. Sen. 1995. *India: Economic Development and Social Opportunity*. New Delhi: Oxford University Press.

Duggal, R. 1997. "Health Care Budgets in a Changing Political Economy." *Economic and Political Weekly*, May 17-24, 1197–1200.

———. 2000. *The Private Health Sector in India: Nature, Trends, and a Critique.* New Delhi: Voluntary Health Association of India.

Duggal, R., S. Nandraj, and A. Vadair. 1995. "Health Expenditures across States, Part II: Regional Disparity in Expenditure." *Economic and Political Weekly*, April 22, 901–08.

Dukes, M.N.G. 2000. "The Reform of the Drug Control System in Uttar Pradesh." Processed.

Eaton, W. W., R. Day, and M. Kramer. 1988. "The Use of Epidemiology for Risk Factor Research in Schizophrenia: An Overview and Methodologic Critique." In M. T. Tsuan and J. C. Simpson, eds., *Handbook of Schizophrenia.* Vol. 3, *Nosology, Epidemiology and Genetics.* Amsterdam: Elsevier Science Publishers.

Ellis, R. P., M. Alam, and I. Gupta. 2000. "Health Insurance in India: Prognosis and Prospectus." *Economic and Political Weekly*, January 22, 207–17.

Francome, C., and W. Savage. 1993. "Caesarean Section in Britain and the United States, 12% or 24%: Is Either the Right Rate?" *Social Science and Medicine* 37:1199–218.

Frank, J. W., and J. F. Mustard. 1994. "The Determinants of Health in a Historical Perspective. *Daedalus* 123(4):1–17.

Frenk, J. 1993. "The Public-Private Mix and Human Resources for Health." *Health Policy and Planning* 8:315–26.

———. 1994. "Dimensions of Health Sector Reform." *Health Policy* 27:19–34.

Garg, C. 2001. "Punjab State Health Accounts." Processed.

Ghosh, A. 1998. "IEC for Promoting Behaviour Change in the Population, Health, and Nutrition Sector, A Review." Paper presented at the workshop on the World Bank's Role in the Health System of India, New Delhi, April 2–3, 1998. Processed.

Girishankar, N. 1999. "Reforming Institutions for Service Delivery: A Framework for Development Assistance with an Application to the HNP Portfolio." Policy Research Working Paper 2039. World Bank, Washington, D.C.

Government of India. 1998–99. "National Health Policy." New Delhi, India.

Greenhalgh, T. 1986. Drug Marketing in the Third World: Beneath the Cosmetic Reforms. *Lancet* 1(8493):1318–20.

Gribble, J. N., and S. H. Preston, eds. 1993. *The Epidemiological Transition.* Washington, D.C.: National Academy Press.

Gupta, R., V. P. Gupta, and N. S. Ahluwalia. 1994. "Educational Status, Coronary Heart Disease, and Coronary Risk Factor Prevalence in a Rural Population of India." *British Medical Journal* 3099:1332–36.

Gwatkin, D., S. Rutstein, K. Johnson, R. P. Pande, and A. Wagstaff. 2000. "Socio-economic Differences in Health, Nutrition, and Population in India." HNP Publication Series, HNP/Poverty Thematic Group. World Bank, Washington, D.C.

Homan, R. K., and K. R. Thankappan. 1999. "An Examination of Public and Private Sector Sources of Inpatient Care in Trivandrum District, Kerala (India) 1999." Kerala: Achuta Menon Center for Health Services. Processed.

IIPS (Indian Institute for Population Sciences). 1995. *National Family Health Survey (MCH and Family Planning), India, 1992–93.* Bombay.

———. 1998–99. *Reproductive and Child Health Surveys.* Bombay.

———. 2000. *National Family Health Survey Summary, India 1998–99.* Bombay.

Institute of Health Systems. 2000. "APVVP Patient Satisfaction Survey 2000." Report Series. Hyderabad.

Kakwani, N., A. Wagstaff, and E. van Doorslaer. 1997. "Socioeconomic Inequalities in Health: Meaurement, Computation, and Statistical Inference." *Journal of Econometrics* 77:87–103.

Kannan, K. P., K. R. Thankappan, V. R. Kutty, and K. P. Aravindan. 1991. "Health and Development in Rural Kerala." Kerala Sastra Sahitya Parishad, Thiruvananthapuram. Processed.

Kathuria, S., and J. Hanson, eds. 2000. *India: Reducing Poverty, Accelerating Development.* New Delhi: Oxford University Press.

Krishnan, T. N. 1995. "Access and the Burden of Treatment: An Inter-State Comparison." Centre for Development Studies. Thiruvananthapuram, Kerala. Processed.

Kumar, D., and R. B. Patel. 1992. "Study of Knowledge, Assessment and Practice of ISM Practitioners and Health Functionaries in the Context of Delivery of MTP Services in Bihar and Maharashtra." Operations Research Group, Baroda, Gujarat Processed.

Last, J. M. 1995. *A Dictionary of Epidemiology.* New York: Oxford University Press.

Mahal, A., V. Srivastava, and D. Sanan. 2001. "Decentralisation and Public Service Delivery in Health and Education Services: Evidence from Rural India." In J.-J. Dethier, ed., *Governance, Decentralization and Reform in China, India and Russia.* Boston: Kluwer Academic Publishers.

Management Sciences for Health. 1997. *Managing Drug Supply: The Selection, Procurement, Distribution, and Use of Pharmaceuticals,* 2nd ed. Bloomfield, Conn.: Kumarian Press.

Mathiyazhagan, K. 1998. "Willingness to Pay for Rural Health Insurance through Community Participation in India." *International Journal of Health Planning and Management* 13:47–67.

Ministry of Health and Family Welfare. 2000a. "Bulletin on Rural Health Statistics in India." Rural Health Division, New Delhi.

———. 2000b. *The National Population Policy 2000.* New Delhi.

Mukhopadhyay, M., ed. 1997. *Report of the Independent Commission on Health in India.* New Delhi: Voluntary Health Association of India Press.

Muraleedharan, V. R. 1997. "Hospital Services in Urban Tamil Nadu: A Survey of Maternity Services in Madras City and Chidambaram/Cuddalore Region." Report prepared for Citizen, Consumer and Civic Action Group, Chennai.

———. 1999a. "Availability and Distribution of Medical, Dental, Nursing and Pharmaceutical Professionals in Tamil Nadu : A Preliminary Assessment." Report submitted to the Tamil Nadu Dr. M. G. R. Medical University, Chennai.

———. 1999b. "Characteristics and Structure of the Private Hospital Sector in Urban India: A Study of Madras City." Small Applied Research Paper 5. Partnerships for Health Reform Project. Bethesda, Md.: Abt Associates.

Murray, C. J. L., and A. D. Lopez. 1996. *The Global Burden of Disease.* Cambridge, Mass.: Harvard University Press.

Musgrove, P. 1999. "Public Spending on Health Care: How Are Different Criteria Related." *Health Policy* 47(3):207–223.

Nandraj, S., and R. Duggal. 1996. "Physical Standards in the Private Health Sector." *Radical Journal of Health* 2(2/3):141–84.

Nandraj, S., A. Khot, and S. Menon. 1999. *Accreditation of Hospitals: Breaking Boundaries in Health Care.* Mumbai: CEHAT.

Narayan, D., R. Chambers, M. K. Sha, and P. Petesch. 2000. *Voices of the Poor: Crying Out for Change*. New York: Oxford University Press.

National Sample Survey Organisation (NSSO). 1992. "Morbidity and Utilisation of Medical Services: NSS 42nd Round (July 1986–June 1987)." *Sarvekshana* 15(4):50–75, S131-S571.

———. 1998. "Morbidity and Treatment of Ailments: NSS Fifty-second Round (July 1995–June 1996)." Calcutta.

OECD (Organisation for Economic Co-operation and Development). 1992. *The Reform of Health Care: A Comparative Analysis of Seven OECD Countries*. Paris.

———. 1994. *The Reform of Health Care Systems: A Review of Seventeen Countries*. Paris.

Osborn, D., and T. Gaebler. 1993. *Reinventing Government*. Reading, Mass.: Addison Wesley.

Pai, M., P. Sundaram, K. K. Radhakrishnan, K. Thomas, and J. P. Muliyil. 1999. "A High Rate of Caesarean Sections in an Affluent Section of Chennai: Is It Cause for Concern? *National Medical Journal of India* 12(4):156–58.

Pauchari, S., ed. 1994. *Reaching India's Poor: Non-governmental Approaches to Community Health*. New Delhi: Sage Publications.

Phadke, A. 1998. *Drug Supply and Use: Towards a Rational Policy in India*. New Delhi: Sage Publications.

Planning Commission. 1998. *Ninth Five-Year Plan 1997–2002*. Vol. II. New Delhi.

Prabhakaran, D., P. Shah, U. Shrivastava, A. K. Prabhakar, B. Shah, V. K. Bahl, S. K. Puri, A. Bhaniani, M. Joshi, and K. S. Reddy. 2000. "Tobacco Consumption in North Indian Males Is Inversely Related to Professional Status: Results of Three Cross Sectional Surveys." Abstract 225/14. 11th World Conference on Tobacco or Health, August 6–11, Chicago.

Preker, A. S., A. Harding, and N. Girishankar. 1999. "The Economics of Private Participation in Health Care: New Insights from Institutional Economics." Paper submitted to the International Social Security Association. Processed.

Preker, A. S., A. Harding, and P. Travis. 2000. "'Make or Buy' Decisions in the Production of Health Care Goods and Services: New Insights from Institutional Economics and Organizational Theory." *Bulletin of the World Health Organization* 78:779–90.

Purohit, B. C. 1995. "Private Voluntary Health Sector in India." *Asian Economic Review* 37:297–311.

Ranson, K. 1999. "The Consequences of Health Insurance for the Informal Sector: Two Non-Governmental, Non-Profit Schemes in Gujarat." London School of Hygiene and Tropical Medicine, Health Policy Unit.

Rao, K. S., G. V. N. Ramana, and H. V. V. Murthy. 1997. "Financing of Primary Health Care in Andhra Pradesh: A Policy Perspective." Administrative Staff College of India, Hyderabad. Processed.

Rao, V. M., N. Alakh, R. Sharma, U. Shrivastava. 1999. *Voices of the Poor: Poverty in People's Perceptions in India.* New Delhi: Institute for Human Development.

Reddy, K. N., and V. Selvaraju. 1994. *Health Care Expenditure by Government of India: 1974–75 to 1990–91.* New Delhi: Seven Hills Publications.

Reddy, K. S., D. Prabhakaran, P. Shah, U. Shrivastava, A. K. Prabhakar, B. Shah, V. K. Bahl, S. K. Puri, A. Bhaniani, and M. Joshi. 2000. "Tobacco Consumption in North Indian Males Is Inversely Related to Educational Level: Results of Three Cross Sectional Surveys." Abstract 225/12. 11th World Conference on Tobacco or Health, August 6–11, Chicago.

Registrar General. Various years. *Sample Registration System Bulletin.* Ministry of Home Affairs, New Delhi.

———. 1995. "Sample Registration System." Ministry of Home Affairs, New Delhi.

———. 1998. *Sample Registration System Bulletin.* October. Ministry of Home Affairs, New Delhi.

———. 1999a. *Compendium of India's Fertility and Mortality Indicators 1971-1997: Based on the Sample Registration System (SRS).* New Delhi.

———. 1999b. *Sample Registration System Bulletin.* April. Ministry of Home Affairs, New Delhi.

———. 2000. *Sample Registration System Bulletin.* April. Ministry of Home Affairs, New Delhi.

Robinson, M. 1997. "Physician-Hospital Integration and Economic Theory of the Firm." *Medical Care Research and Review* 54:1.

Roemer, M. I. 1991. *National Health Systems of the World.* 2 vols. New York: Oxford University Press.

Rohde, J., and H. Viswanathan. 1995. *The Rural Private Practitioner*. New Delhi: Oxford University Press.

Saltman, R. B., and O. Ferroussier-David. 2000. "On the Concept of Stewardship in Health Policy." *Bulletin of the World Health Organization* 78:732–39.

Saltman, R. B., and J. Figueras. 1998. "Analyzing the Evidence on European Health Care Reforms. *Health Affairs (Millwood)* 17(2):85–108.

———. eds. 1997. *European Health Care Reform: Analysis of Current Strategies*. Eurpoean Series 72. Copenhagen: WHO Regional Office for Europe.

Satia, J. 1999. "Institutional Assessment: Strengthening Routine Immunization— India." World Bank, New Delhi. Processed.

Selvaraju, V. 2000. "Public Expenditures on Health in India." Background paper for National Council of Applied Economic Research. Processed.

Sen, P. 1997. "Community Control of Health Financing in India: A Review of Local Experiences." Bethesda, Md.: Abt Associates.

Shah, G. 1996. "Public Health—Urban Society Interface: A Study of Pneumonic Plague in Surat." Centre for Social Studies, Surat, Gujarat. Processed.

Shariff, A. 1997. "Human Development Profile of Rural India: Inter-State and Inter-Group Differentials: A Summary." NCAER, New Delhi.

Sharma, S., W. McGreevey, and D. Hotchkiss. 2000. "Financing Reproductive and Child Health Care in Rajasthan." USAID Report, Indian Institute for Health Management Research, The Policy Project, The Futures Group. New Delhi.

Stafford, R. S. 1990. "Cesarean Section Use and Source of Payment: An Analysis of Canadian Hospital Discharge Abstracts." *American Journal of Public Health* 80:313–15.

STEM (Center for Symbiosis of Technology, Environment and Management). 2000. "Uttar Pradesh Health Systems Development Project: Baseline Study." Project Report. Bangalore, Karnataka.

Thaver, I. H., T. Harpham, B. McPake, and P. Garner. 1998. "Private Practitioners in the Slums of Karachi: What Quality of Care Do They Offer?" *Social Science and Medicine* 46:1441–9

Tulasidhar, V. B. 1992. *State's Financing of Health Care in India: Some Recent Trends*. New Delhi: National Institute of Public Finance and Policy.

———. 1996. "Government Health Expenditures in India: Public Financing for Health in India: Recent Trends." Supported by the International Health Policy Program. Processed.

Upleker, M. W., and D. S. Shepard. 1991. *Treatment of Tuberculosis by Private General Practitioners in India*. Bombay: Foundation for Research in Community Health.

U.S. Department of Health and Human Services. 1991. *Healthy People 2000*. DHHS Publication No. (PHS) 91-50212, Washington, D.C.

Wagstaff, A. 2002. "Inequality Aversion, Health Inequalities and Health Achievement." Policy Research Working Paper 2765. World Bank, Policy Research Department, Washington D.C.

Wang, J., D. T. Jamison, E. Bos, A. S. Preker, J. Peadbody. 1999. *Measuring Country Performance on Health: Selected Indicators for 115 Countries*. Health, Nutrition, and Population Series. Washington, D.C.: World Bank.

WHO (World Health Organization). 1985. "Appropriate Technology for Birth." *Lancet* 2(8452):436–37.

———. 1995. "The Treatment of Diarrhoea: A Manual for Physicians and other Senior Health Workers." WHO/CDR/95.3. Geneva .

———. 1999. *World Health Report 1999: Making a Difference*. Geneva.

———. 2000a. *Health a Key to Prosperity: Success Stories in Developing Countries*. Geneva.

———. 2000b. "Research into Action." Report on Tuberculosis Research. Regional Office for South-East Asia.

———. 2000c. *World Health Report 2000: Health Systems: Improving Performance*. Geneva.

———. 2001. *Involving Private Practitioners in Tuberculosis Control: Issues, Interventions, and Emerging Policy Framework*. Geneva.

World Bank. 1993. *World Development Report 1993: Investing in Health*. New York: Oxford University Press.

———. 1995. "India: Policy and Finance Strategies for Strengthening Primary Health Care Services." Report 13042-IN. Washington, D.C.

———. 1996. "Staff Appraisal Report: State Health Systems Development Project II." Report 15106-IN. Washington, D.C.

———. 1997a. "Health, Nutrition, and Population: Sector Strategy." Health, Nutrition, Population Department. Washington, D.C.

———. 1997b. "India: New Directions in Health Sector Development at the State Level: An Operational Perspective." Report 15753-IN. Washington, D.C.

———. 1997c. "Project Appraisal Document: Malaria Control Project." Report 16393-IN. Washington, D.C.

———. 1999a. *Curbing the Epidemic: Governments and the Economics of Tobacco Control.* Development in Practice Series. Washington, D.C.

———. 1999b. "India Second State Health Systems Project, Mid-Term Review Report." South Asia Region. Washington, D.C.

———. 2000a. "Confronting Poverty: The Challenge of Uttar Pradesh." South Asia Region. Washington, D.C.

———. 2000b. *Poverty Reduction Strategy Sourcebook* (CD-ROM). Poverty Reduction Economic Management, Poverty Unit. Washington D.C. Also available at http://www.worldbank.org/poverty/strategies/sourctoc.htm

———. 2000c. "Project Appraisal Document. Immunization Strengthening Project." Report 19894-IN. Washington, D.C.

———. 2000d. *World Development Indicators.* New York: Oxford University Press.

———. 2000e. *World Development Report 2000/2001: Attacking Poverty.* New York: Oxford University Press.

———. 2001. "Project Appraisal Document. Second National Leprosy Elimination Project." Report 21751-IN. Washington, D.C.

Yaqub, S. 1999. "How Equitable is Public Spending on Health and Education." Background paper to World Bank (2000c).

Yesudian, C. A. K. 1994. "The Behaviour of the Private Sector in the Health Service Market of Bombay." *Health Policy Planning* 9(1):72–80.